Oncology

International Journal of Cancer Research and Treatment

Founded 1948 as 'Oncologia' by H.R. Schinz
Continued by V. Richards (1967–1975), H. Wrba (1976–1992)

KARGER

Printed in Switzerland
on acid-free paper by
Reinhardt Druck, Basel

Appears 6-weekly:
2 volumes per year
(8 issues)

Guidelines for Authors

Oncology

Submission

Only original papers written in English are considered and should be sent to:

Prof. P.P. Carbone
S. Karger AG
Editorial Office Oncology
P.O. Box
CH–4009 Basel (Switzerland)
Tel. +41 61 306 1359
Fax +41 61 306 1434
E-Mail k.tschopp@karger.ch

Mailing address for courier deliveries only:
Allschwilerstr. 10
CH–4055 Basel (Switzerland)

Manuscripts should be submitted in quadruplicate (with four sets of illustrations), typewritten double-spaced on one side of the paper, with a wide margin. The final version of your manuscript and illustrations should also be submitted on disk. For details refer to 'Disk Submission' or www.karger.com/journals/disksub.htm. Editorial review and copy-editing will be executed from the disk version of your manuscript. Names and addresses of four experts in the appropriate area of research should accompany each manuscript. Selected scientist(s) will be invited to act as referee(s). Referees suggested should not be from the same institution as the author and should have expert knowledge of the subject.

Conditions

All manuscripts are subject to editorial review. The editors reserve the right to improve style and, if necessary, return the manuscript for rewriting to the author. Submission of an article for publication implies the transfer of the copyright from the author to the publisher upon acceptance. Accepted papers become the permanent property of 'Oncology' and may not be reproduced by any means, in whole or in part, without the written consent of the publisher. It is the author's responsibility to obtain permission to reproduce illustrations, tables, etc. from other publications.

All manuscripts originating from non-English speaking countries must be revised by a professional linguistic reviewer and it must be evident from the covering letter that this has been done.

The editor reserves the right to reject papers based on priorities and space availability in the journal.

Arrangement

Title page: The first page of each paper should indicate the title (main title underlined), the authors' names, and the institute where the work was conducted. A short title for use as running head as well as the full address of the author to whom correspondence should be sent are also required.

Full address: The exact postal address complete with postal code must be given at the bottom of the title page. Please also supply phone and fax numbers, as well as your e-mail address.

Key words: For indexing purposes, a list of 3–10 key words in English is essential.

Abstract: **Each paper needs an abstract of up to 200 words. Abstracts of papers submitted for publication that have clinical implications using human materials should be structured with subheadings as follows: Objective(s), Methods, Results, Conclusion(s).**

Small type: Paragraphs which can or must be set in smaller type (case histories, test methods, etc.) should be indicated with a 'p' (petit) in the margin on the left-hand side.

Footnotes: Avoid footnotes. When essential, they are numbered consecutively and typed at the foot of the appropriate page.

Tables and illustrations: Tables and illustrations (both numbered in Arabic numerals) should be prepared on separate sheets. Tables require a heading and figures a legend, also prepared on a separate sheet. For the reproduction of illustrations, only good drawings and original photographs can be accepted; negatives or photocopies cannot be used. Due to technical reasons, figures with a screen background should not be submitted. When possible, group several illustrations on one block for reproduction (max. size 181 × 223 mm) or provide crop marks. On the back of each illustration, indicate its number, the author's name, and 'top' with a soft pencil.

Color illustrations: Up to 6 color illustrations per page can be integrated within the text at the reduced price of CHF 660.–/USD 545.00 per page. Color illustrations are reproduced at the author's expense.

References: In the text identify references by Arabic numerals [in square brackets]. Material submitted for publication but not yet accepted should be noted as 'unpublished data' and not be included in the reference list. The list of references should include only those publications which are cited in the text. Do not alphabetize; number references in the order in which they are first mentioned in the text. The surnames of the authors followed by initials should be given. There should be no punctuation other than a comma to separate the authors. Cite all authors, 'et al' is not sufficient. Abbreviate journal names according to the Index Medicus system. (Also see International Committee of Medical Journal Editors: Uniform requirements for manuscripts submitted to biomedical journals. N Engl J Med 1997;336:309–315.)

Examples

(a) Papers published in periodicals: Sun J, Koto H, Chung KF: Interaction of ozone and allergen challenges on bronchial responsiveness and inflammation in sensitised guinea pigs. Int Arch Allergy Immunol 1997;112:191–195.

(b) Monographs: Matthews DE, Farewell VT: Using and Understanding Medical Statistics, ed 3, revised. Basel, Karger, 1996.

(c) Edited books: Parren PWHI, Burton DR: Antibodies against HIV-1 from phage display libraries: Mapping of an immune response and progress towards antiviral immunotherapy; in Capra JD (ed): Antibody Engineering. Chem Immunol. Basel, Karger, 1997, vol 65, pp 18–56.

(d) Papers published in electronic format: Black CA: Delayed type hypersensitivity: Current theories with a historic perspective. Dermatol Online J 1999;5:7. http://dermatology.cdlib.org/DOJvol5num1.

Page charges

There are no page charges for papers of 3 or fewer printed pages (including tables, illustrations and references). Each additional complete or partial page is charged to the author at CHF 275.– / USD 196.00. The allotted size of a paper is equal to approx. 9 manuscript pages (including tables, illustrations and references).

Galley proofs

Unless indicated otherwise, galley proofs are sent to the first-named author and should be returned with the least possible delay. Alterations made in galley proofs, other than the correction of printer's errors, are charged to the author. No page proofs are supplied.

Reprints

Order forms and a price list are sent with the galley proofs. Orders submitted after the issue is printed are subject to considerably higher prices.

KARGER

Fax +41 61 306 12 34
E-Mail karger@karger.ch
www.karger.com

The Guidelines for Authors are available at:
www.karger.com/journals/ocl/ocl_gl.htm

Oncology

General Information

Publication data: 'Oncology' is published 8 times a year. Volumes 60–61, each with 4 issues, appear in 2001.

Subscription rates: Subscriptions run for a full calendar year. Prices are given per volume.
Personal subscription:
Subscription + postage and handling
CHF 358.– + CHF 18.25 Europe
CHF 358.– + CHF 27.20 Overseas
USD 275.50 + USD 18.25
+ online subscription per volume:
CHF 39.– / USD 30.00
(Must be in the name of, billed to, and paid by an individual. Order must be marked 'personal subscription'.)
Institutional subscription:
Subscription + postage and handling
CHF 716.– + CHF 22.80 Europe
CHF 716.– + CHF 34.– Overseas
USD 551.00 + USD 22.80
+ online subscription per volume:
CHF 58.– / USD 45.00
Airmail postage: CHF 24.–, USD 20.00.
(Extra per volume.)

Microforms: Please direct all enquiries and orders to: University Microfilms Inc.
300 North Zeeb Road, P.O. Box 1346
Ann Arbor, MI 48106-1346 (USA)

Advertising: Correspondence and rate requests should be addressed to the Publisher.

Subscription orders: Orders can be placed at agencies, bookstores, directly with the Publisher
S. Karger AG, P.O. Box,
CH–4009 Basel (Switzerland)
or with any of the following distributors:
Deutschland: S. Karger GmbH, Postfach
D–79095 Freiburg
France: Librairie Luginbühl
36, bd de Latour-Maubourg, F–75007 Paris
Great Britain, Ireland: S. Karger Publishers
58 Grove Hill Road
Tunbridge Wells, Kent TN1 1SP, UK
USA: S. Karger Publishers, Inc.
26 West Avon Road, P.O. Box 529
Farmington, CT 06085, USA
India, Bangladesh, Sri Lanka:
Panther Publishers Private Ltd.
39, 6th Cross
Wilson Gardens
Bangalore 560 027, India
Japan: Katakura Libri, Inc.
2F, Marushima Bldg, 4-6-17, Yushima,
Bunkyo-ku, Tokyo 113-0034, Japan

Change of address: Both old and new address should be sent to the subscription source.

Single issues and back volumes: Information can be obtained through the Publisher.

Bibliographic indices: This journal is regularly listed in bibliographic services, including *Current Contents®*.

Book Reviews: Books are accepted for review by special agreement.

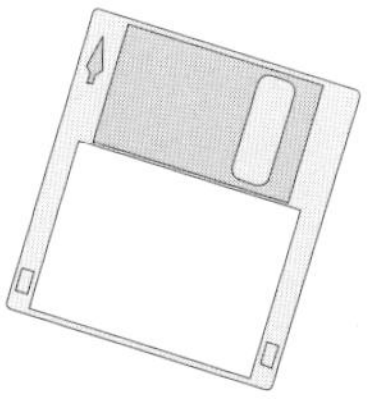

Disk Submission

A **comprehensive version** of these guidelines for the **submission of manuscripts and illustrations on disk** can be accessed online under **www.karger.com/journals/disksub.htm** or requested as a leaflet from the editorial department.

Please follow the general rules on style and arrangement in the **'Guidelines for Authors'** of the journal. Submit a **double-spaced printout** of your manuscript matching the file on disk exactly.

Technical Information

Store only data pertinent to this manuscript. Include your fonts (screen and printer fonts for Macintosh). For a **text only** manuscript, use a 3.5-inch disk. For **text and illustrations,** use 3.5 or 5.25 Magneto Optical Disc; CD-ROM (DOS or hybrid); iomage Zip/DOS (100 MB), or 44 MB, 88 MB or 200 MB SyQuest. Compress extensive data using ZIP format.

Data Description

Label your disk with the **title of the journal or book** for which it is submitted; a **short version** of the paper's title; your **name,** postal and e-mail address, fax and phone number; **hard- and software** used, including the version; and the **complete list of the file names.** File names consist of eight characters before the dot identifying the file and three characters after the dot identifying the application.

Text and Format

The **preferred word-processing package is MS-Word.** Other commonly used PC text programs and ASCII formats are accepted.
Update your data when you revise subsequent to the reviewer's or editor's decision and mark revisions clearly. Manuscripts accepted for publication are subject to **copy editing:** changes and/or questions will be marked in the manuscript, which will be returned to you with your disk and the galley proofs for checking.
Enter your text continuously flush left. Do not use any layout functions. Do not split words at the end of a line. **Do not use indentations.** Use a blank line before and a hard return at the end of paragraphs. **Arrange headings flush left.** Insert only **one space after punctuation marks.** Insert Greek letters, mathematical symbols etc. with your word-processing program. Use **boldface and italics** as well as sub- and superscript where appropriate.
Tables are part of the text and should be placed at the end of the text file. Separate the individual parts of a table by lines. Use the tabulator instead of spaces. Format operation data on one line in the same column. **Legends to illustrations are part of the text** and should also be listed at the end of the text file.

Illustrations

Store illustrations as separate files: do not integrate them in your text. Export **line drawings/vector graphics** as TIF, EPS or WMF format. Use Photoshop for processing and retouching **scanned halftone images.** Save the original scan and the processed version. Export **black and white or color images** as TIF or EPS format in their anticipated size in print. **For detailed information** on how to submit illustration data on disk please consult the leaflet or **www.karger.com/journals/disksub.htm.**

KARGER

Fax +41 61 306 12 34
E-Mail karger@karger.ch
www.karger.com

The Journal Home Page is available at:
www.karger.com/journals/ocl

KI 98 DISK

Oncology

Optimising the Role of Herceptin® in Breast Cancer

Proceedings of a Symposium, Monte Carlo, June 19–21, 2000

Guest Editor
David Khayat, Paris, France

KARGER

Basel · Freiburg · Paris · London · New York ·
New Delhi · Bangkok · Singapore · Tokyo · Sydney

Supported by an educational grant from F. Hoffmann-La Roche Ltd, Basel, Switzerland

The opinions and views expressed in this educational supplement are those of the authors and do not necessarily reflect the opinions or recommendations of F. Hoffmann-La Roche Ltd. The articles in this supplement may discuss uses and dosages of Herceptin or other pharmaceutical agents that are not approved by regulatory authorities in Europe and elsewhere. Please consult local prescribing information before using any product.

S. Karger
Medical and Scientific Publishers
Basel · Freiburg · Paris · London
New York · New Delhi · Bangkok
Singapore · Tokyo · Sydney

Drug Dosage
The authors and the publisher have exerted every effort to ensure that drug selection and dosage set forth in this text are in accord with current recommendations and practice at the time of publication. However, in view of ongoing research, changes in government regulations, and the constant flow of information relating to drug therapy and drug reactions, the reader is urged to check the package insert for each drug for any change in indications and dosage and for added warnings and precautions. This is particularly important when the recommended agent is a new and/or infrequently employed drug.

P.O. Box, CH–4009 Basel (Switzerland)
Printed in Switzerland on acid-free paper by
Reinhardt Druck, Basel
ISBN 3–8055–7327–8

KARGER

Fax + 41 61 306 12 34
E-Mail karger@karger.ch
www.karger.com

Vol. 61, Suppl. 2, 2001

Oncology

Contents

KARGER

Fax + 41 61 306 12 34
E-Mail karger@karger.ch
www.karger.com

Access to full text and tables of contents, including tentative ones for forthcoming issues:
www.karger.com/journals/ocl/ocl_bk.htm

Oncology

Preface

Therapeutic interventions for cancer, including surgery, radiotherapy and chemotherapy, generally have limited specificity and cause considerable toxicity due to their effects on normal cells. This often limits their usefulness and acceptability. and can result in less than optimal treatment of patients with cancer. Therefore, tumor-specific therapy has been of considerable interest for many years, although until relatively recently hormonal therapy was the only targeted therapy shown to have anticancer activity.

Over the past 20–30 years, our understanding of how tumors develop has advanced considerably and tumors are recognised to be the result of the accumulation of mutations affecting intrinsic processes controlling cell growth, differentiation and survival. This recognition has caused a revolution in therapeutic development, with agents being developed to specifically target and inhibit abnormal cellular factors and processes. The expectation that these agents would have efficacy and reduced toxicity has been fulfilled by the first targeted agents to be developed, MabThera® and Herceptin®.

The humanized monoclonal antibody Herceptin targets human epidermal growth factor receptor-2 (HER2) positive cells, i.e. cells in which HER2 is amplified/overexpressed, a feature associated with many tumor characteristics. Approximately 20–30% of breast cancers are HER2 positive and are known to be particularly aggressive. Thus, HER2-positive cancer constitutes a rational target for therapy. Clinical trials of Herceptin have clearly demonstrated that it provides significant clinical benefit in HER2-positive metastatic disease, most importantly increased survival when administered first line in combination with chemotherapy. Furthermore, Herceptin is generally well tolerated, with none of the side effects typical of chemotherapy. The articles in this supplement review our knowledge of the activity of HER2 and how to test for HER2 status use, and describe the clinical trials of Herceptin that have been performed to date.

Herceptin is now an established therapy for HER2-positive metastatic breast cancer and is approved for use first line in combination with paclitaxel and second/third line as a single agent. However, research to optimize the use of Herceptin continues.

It is widely believed that increasing tumor characterization will result in increasingly individualized anticancer therapy. Important lessons can be learned from the process of establishing how to test for HER2 and what constitutes a positive result. These lessons possibly include ensuring that the test used in clinical trials can be used generally and ensuring that test results are clinically relevant.

Agents such as Herceptin also require a change in our thinking about how to use drug therapy. Thus, Herceptin can be used for extended periods rather than a fixed number of cycles due to its tolerability and continued growth-suppressing effects on tumor cells. The implications of this are that it is possible that Herceptin can be administered beyond initial disease progression, while the combination agent is changed. In addition, the optimal Herceptin-containing combination is likely to vary between patients due to differing tumor characteristics and drug interactions. Finally, early use of Herceptin, when tumor burden is least, is likely to be most effective. This has been clearly demonstrated in the metastatic setting and is now being extended into the adjuvant and neoadjuvant settings in clinical trials.

In conclusion, while Herceptin has already stimulated a dramatic change in how therapy is developed and expectations of new therapies, future research with this novel agent is likely to change how we manage cancer patients and further improve the efficacy of therapy.

David Khayat

KARGER

Fax + 41 61 306 12 34
E-Mail karger@karger.ch
www.karger.com

Accessible online at:
www.karger.com/journals/ocl

Oncology

Oncology 2001;61(suppl 2):1–13

Biology of HER2 and Its Importance in Breast Cancer

Yosef Yarden

Department of Biological Regulation, The Weizmann Institute of Science, Rehovot, Israel

Key Words
HER2 (erbB-2, *neu*) · Receptor · Tumor growth · Breast cancer · Monoclonal antibody · Herceptin® · Trastuzumab · Network · Signaling

Abstract
Human epidermal growth factor receptor-2 (HER2/erbB-2) belongs to a family of four transmembrane receptors involved in signal transduction pathways that regulate cell growth and differentiation. Overexpression/amplification of HER2 is associated with malignancy and a poor prognosis in breast cancer. HER2 acts as a networking receptor that mediates signaling to cancer cells, causing them to proliferate. HER receptors exist as monomers but dimerize on ligand binding. HER ligands are bivalent growth factor molecules whose low-affinity site binds to HER2. No HER2-specific ligand has been identified but HER2 is the preferred heterodimerization partner for other HER receptors. HER2-containing heterodimers are relatively long-lived and potent. HER3 has no inherent activity and is the major and most potent dimerization partner of HER2. HER2 overexpression biases the formation of HER2-containing heterodimers, leading to enhanced responsiveness to stromal growth factors and oncogenic transformation. Removal of HER2 from the cell surface or inhibition of its intrinsic enzymatic activity may reduce oncogenicity. Our research suggests that the antitumor efficacy of HER2-specific antibodies such as Herceptin® relates to their ability to direct HER2 to a Cbl-dependent endocytosis and degradation pathway. The reported clinical therapeutic efficacy of anti-HER2 monoclonal antibodies in breast cancer highlights the importance of understanding the biology of HER2.

Introduction

Human epidermal growth factor receptor-2 (HER2) is the second member of the human epidermal growth factor receptor (HER) family [Hung and Lau 1999]. It plays a key role in the HER family, cooperating with other HER receptors via a complex signaling network to regulate cell growth, differentiation and survival. The HER2 proto-oncogene (also known as *neu* or c-*erb*B-2) encodes the transmembrane HER2 protein. HER2 is normally expressed in a variety of cell and tissue types excluding those of hematopoietic origin [Hynes and Stern 1994], and, importantly, is frequently overexpressed in a number of human cancers. Although HER2 is widely distributed, its signaling activity is regulated by the presence of HER agonists (ligands) and transmodulating partners [Hynes and Stern 1994].

The HER receptor family is involved in the regulation of normal breast growth and development [Carraway et al. 1997], and overexpression of HER2 is associated with cancer of the breast [Slamon et al. 1989]. HER2 gene amplification (generation of more than the normal two gene copies) is the most common mechanism leading to

KARGER

Fax + 41 61 306 12 34
E-Mail karger@karger.ch
www.karger.com

0030–2414/01/0616–0001$17.50/0

Accessible online at:
www.karger.com/journals/ocl

Y. Yarden, PhD
Department of Biological Regulation, The Weizmann Institute of Science
Rehovot, 76100 (Israel)
Tel. +972 8 934 3974, Fax +972 8 934 2488
E-Mail yosef.yarden@weizmann.ac.il

increased HER2 protein expression [Hynes and Stern 1994]. Amplification of the HER2 gene leads to overexpression of the receptor and disrupts normal control mechanisms, potentially leading to the formation of aggressive tumor cells [Hung et al. 1986].

HER2 amplification was first noted in human breast cancer and was subsequently identified in ovarian cancer [Berchuck et al. 1990; Slamon et al. 1987, 1989; Zhang et al. 1989]. The HER2 gene is amplified in approximately 20 to 30% of breast cancers [McCann et al. 1991; van de Vijver et al. 1987] and is associated with aggressive tumor behavior [Hynes and Stern 1994]. The association between HER2 overexpression and a poor prognosis is supported by the significantly shorter overall survival rate and time to relapse in patients with HER2-overexpressing breast or ovarian cancer relative to patients with tumors without HER2 overexpression [Berchuck et al. 1990; Slamon et al. 1987, 1989]. HER2 overexpression/amplification has also been found in lung, gastric and oral cancers with high frequencies [Hou et al. 1992; Schneider et al. 1989; Weiner et al. 1990; Yokota et al. 1988; Yoshida et al. 1989; Xia et al. 1997].

Breast cancer is currently the most common cancer in women and in Western countries it is the second leading cause of death in women after lung cancer [Devesa et al. 1995; Estéve et al. 1996]. Treatment of breast cancer relies on a multimodality approach, including surgery, radiation, hormone therapy, chemotherapy and supportive therapy. In many cases, especially in advanced disease, the cancer does not respond to conventional treatment. The prognosis of patients with breast carcinoma is primarily dependent on the TNM (tumor, nodes, metastases) stage of the disease. The levels of estrogen receptor and progesterone receptor have prognostic significance for survival and risk of occurrence and are the main predictive indicators of response to hormonal treatment [ASCO 1998]. In metastatic breast cancer, hormonal and chemotherapy are the mainstay of treatment because of the systemic nature of the disease. Currently, metastatic breast cancer remains incurable with a median survival in the range of 17 to 20 months. Therefore, there is an urgent need for new treatment options for this devastating condition.

With regard to the HER2 receptor, the main areas of experimentation and interest are the extent of the involvement of HER2 in the progression of breast carcinoma, the utility of HER2 abnormalities as a prognostic indicator and predictive factor for response to therapy, and the potential use of HER2 as a therapeutic target. In addition to its prognostic value, some evidence is available in support of the ability of HER2 to predict for a resistance to hormonal therapy and some types of cytotoxic chemotherapy [for a review, see Ross and Fletcher 1998; Piccart et al. 2001]. However, interpretation of the current data is complex and no definitive conclusions can be drawn at present.

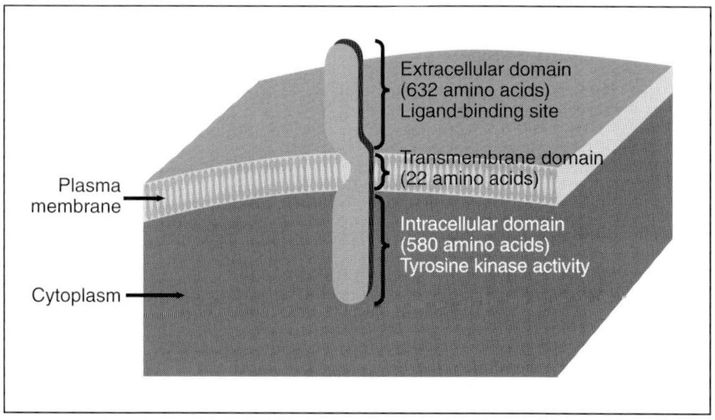

Fig. 1. Structure of the HER2 protein.

Apart from the clinical utility of HER2 in obtaining prognostic and predictive information to guide patient management and treatment selection, the overexpressed HER2 receptor represents an ideal target for specific anticancer therapies. The strategic development of the anti-HER2 monoclonal antibody (MAb), Herceptin® (trastuzumab) is an example of one such HER2-specific therapy. Indeed, research into the biology of the receptor is not only helping to elucidate the mechanism of action of novel anti-HER2 treatments but is also providing new targets for cancer therapy. This review describes the current understanding of the complex HER2 signaling network and how this knowledge is leading to the development of new anticancer therapies that target the HER2 receptor.

The HER Family

The evolution of the HER signaling network has occurred in parallel with that of complex life forms. HER-like receptors are found in the membranes of simpler life forms and ancestral forms of the HER molecule with tyrosine kinase activity are found in invertebrates. For example, the worm *Caenorhabditis elegans* has a single epidermal HER-like receptor that binds only one ligand. The fruit fly *Drosophila melanogaster* also possesses a HER-like receptor, but this binds four growth factors. In contrast, mammals are known to have a family of four closely

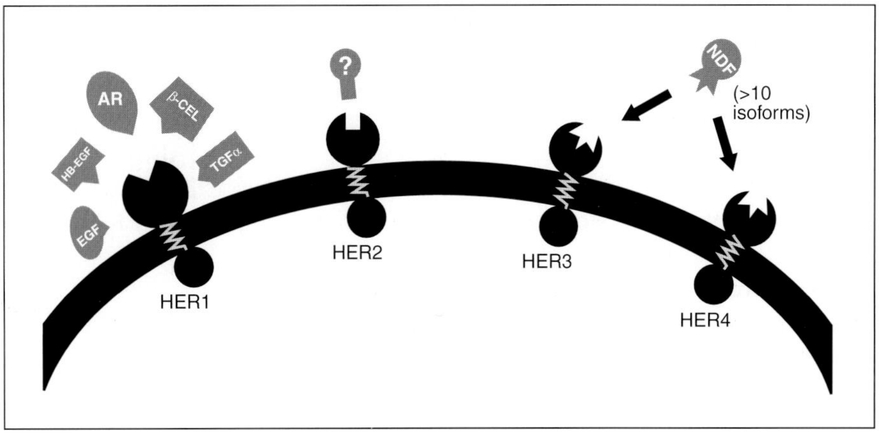

Fig. 2. Mammalian HER family.

related growth factor receptors that bind a variety of ligands, as discussed below.

The HER family comprises four genes encoding four homologous HER receptors [Tzahar et al. 1998]. The receptors are all located on the cell membrane and are found in a variety of tissues. They interact with a range of growth-factor ligands, all of which share an EGF-like motif of 50 to 55 amino acids, including six highly conserved cysteine residues [Akiyama et al. 1986].

The rat *neu* gene was originally isolated from rat neuroblastoma and its normal cellular counterpart was subsequently isolated from rat and human cDNA libraries [Bargmann et al. 1986; Hung et al. 1986; Yamamoto et al. 1986; Coussens et al. 1985]. The various naming systems for these genes are the result of the discovery of homologous genes involved in the pathogenesis of erythroblastoma in chickens (erbB) [Vennstrom and Bishop 1982] and of genes encoding growth factor receptors in humans (HER). However, HER is the most commonly used designation. HER2 is a proto-oncogene mapped to chromosome 17q21. It encodes a 1,255 amino acid transmembrane glycoprotein of molecular weight 185 kDa [Akiyama et al. 1986] designated as $p185^{HER2}$, which is often simply called the HER2 protein or receptor.

Structure of HER Receptors

The four-member HER family of receptors comprises epidermal growth factor receptor (EGFR) or HER1, HER2, HER3 and HER4 [Lupu et al. 1995] [for a review, see Ross and Fletcher 1998]. The HER receptors are located at the cell membrane and share a similar structure, comprising a cysteine-rich extracellular growth factor (ligand) binding domain, a lipophilic transmembrane segment and an intracellular tyrosine kinase domain with a regulatory carboxyl-terminal segment (fig. 1) [van der Geer et al. 1994]. Unlike the other three HER receptors, HER3 fails to conserve certain residues in the catalytic domain that are usually invariant in protein kinases, suggesting that it has weak kinase activity [Hynes and Stern 1994]. Activation of HER receptors via their tyrosine kinase activity results in signal transduction to the nucleus and ultimately leads to nuclear gene activation and cell division.

Role of HER2 in Development

The HER family plays an important role in human development. In human fetuses, HER2 has been detected in the nervous system, developing bone, muscle, skin, heart, lungs and intestinal epithelium [Coussens et al. 1985; Quirke et al. 1989]. One example of the role of HER2 during embryonic development is the indirect binding of the ligand neuregulin-1 to HER2 to control the development of trabeculae in the heart. Growth factor secreted from the endocardium activates the receptor HER2 in combination with HER4 in the myocardium, and this results in formation of trabeculae in the ventricle. Research has shown that if HER2 is absent in the developing mouse embryo, the trabeculae will not form and the mice will die in the uterus during gestation [Meyer and Birchmeyer 1995].

An example of the role of HER2 after birth is its involvement in the regulation of normal breast growth and development. The EGF-like ligands and neuregulins that bind to this receptor family have been shown to stimulate the lobulo-alveolar development of the mouse mammary gland in explant cultures and in vivo [Di Augustine and Richards 1997; Jones et al. 1996; Normanno and Ciardiello 1997; Yang et al. 1995].

Activation of HER Receptors

HER proteins exist as monomers in the plasma membrane. HER activation is usually dependent on the presence of small molecules called ligands [Akiyama et al. 1988; Kokai et al. 1989] and other receptors of the HER family [Connelly and Stern 1990]. Following ligand binding, the four different receptors can associate with each other to form ten different receptor dimers, which may be homodimers (e.g., HER1-HER1) or heterodimers (e.g., HER1-HER2) [Alroy and Yarden 1997]. It is noteworthy that the dimer complex formed between a ligand and two receptors is more stable than a monomeric receptor complex.

The mammalian HER family and its various ligands are illustrated in fig. 2. HER1 binds to several ligands: epidermal growth factor (EGF), transforming growth factor alpha (TGFα), amphiregulin (AR), heparin-binding EGF-like growth factor (HB-EGF), betacellulin (β-cel) and epiregulin. HER2 is shown as not having a known ligand since none has been identified to date. HER3 and HER4 bind to many neuregulins or neu differentiation factors (NDFs), a family of structurally diverse peptides [Alroy and Yarden 1997]. Signaling by all neuregulins is directed through mitogen-activated protein kinase (MAPK) [Pinkas-Kramarski et al. 1996].

Ligand Binding to HER Receptors

Extensive research by several research groups, including ours, has discovered no direct ligand for HER2. However, confirmation of this is expected following completion of the human genome project. Evidence for HER2 being a ligandless receptor has come from our research on pox viruses. The viruses encode EGF-like ligands that interact with the host's HER receptors, causing epithelial lesions. To test whether any of these ligands interact with HER2, we constructed ligands representative of the pox virus growth factors, and tested their binding specificity to receptors in the HER family. Although they interacted with many of the different homodimer and heterodimer combinations of HER family members, none of them

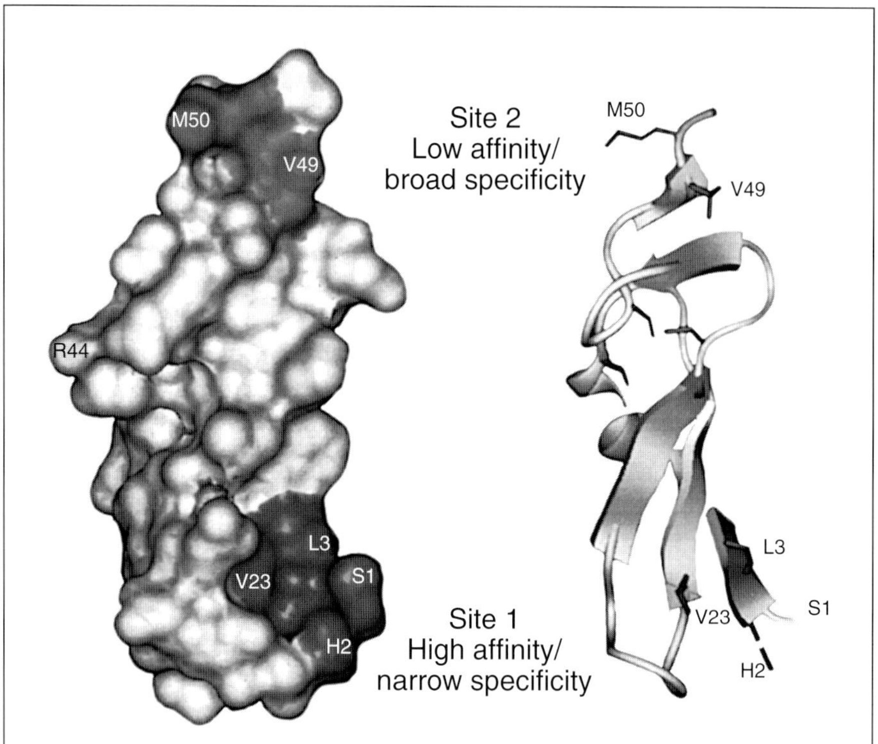

Fig. 3. The 3-D structure of neuregulin-1.

bound with a HER2 homodimer [Klapper et al. 1999]. All were, however, able to recruit HER2 into heterodimers. This led us to propose that HER2 functions as a ligandless receptor for many, if not all, HER ligands [Tzahar et al. 1998].

Although this suggests that HER2 has no ligand of its own, we propose that HER2 acts as a co-receptor, enabling it to heterodimerize and participate in signal transduction in the absence of a specific ligand. Our research with growth factors, such as neuregulin-1, implies that HER ligands are bivalent molecules, i.e. they have two binding sites for HER receptors. Neuregulin-1 has two binding sites for HER proteins: a high-affinity, narrow-specificity site (N-terminal) and a low-affinity, broad-specificity site (C-terminal) [Tzahar et al. 1997] (fig. 3). Significantly, we found that HER2 preferentially binds to the low-affinity site. Our studies suggest that ligands have a high-affinity site that binds directly to the receptor HER1, HER3 or HER4, and a carboxy-terminal, low-affinity site that recruits a homo or heterodimerization partner, which in most cases is HER2 (fig. 4). Significantly, HER2 is a co-receptor for many different ligands and is often transactivated by EGF-like ligands, resulting in the formation of HER1-HER2 heterodimers [Pinkas-Kramarski et al. 1996, 1997]. Neuregulins display greater binding specificity for HER2-HER3 and HER2-HER4 heterodimers [Pinkas-Kramarski et al. 1998; Baly et al. 1997; Burden and Yarden 1997; Tzahar et al. 1996]. Indeed, interactions within the HER family do not occur at random. Rather, there is a clear hierarchy that prefers HER2 as a dimerization partner.

It appears, therefore, that HER2 developed as a low-affinity receptor for many ligands that share the bivalent structure. Importantly, heterodimerization enables HER2 to act as a co-receptor and participate in signal transduction in the absence of a specific ligand. Overexpression of HER2 in human cancer cells enhances this preferential binding of the low-affinity arm of ligands to HER2 and results in increased intracellular signaling [Tzahar and Yarden 1998]. This mechanism appears to be a critical part of the oncogenesis model.

In order to analyze the interactions between the individual HER family members and ligands, we created a cellular system comprising the interleukin-3-dependent myeloid 32D cell line. Transfecting the various HER receptors into the 32D cells generated the corresponding cell lines, D1, D2, D3 and D4. In the absence of interleukin-3, D1 cells grew in the presence of EGF or TGF-α. However, D2 cells did not survive in the presence of any of these ligands, implying that HER2 has no direct ligand. This is also found to be the case with D3 cells because HER3 does not have an inherent kinase activity.

When we created cell lines that co-expressed two receptors, e.g. D1–2 cells expressing the HER1 and HER2 receptors, we obtained predictable results. The most significant observation was noted with the combination of HER2 and HER3 in D2–3 cells. Figure 5 illustrates the results of such mitogenic activity tests. The tests showed that HER1 homodimers are relatively weak signaling

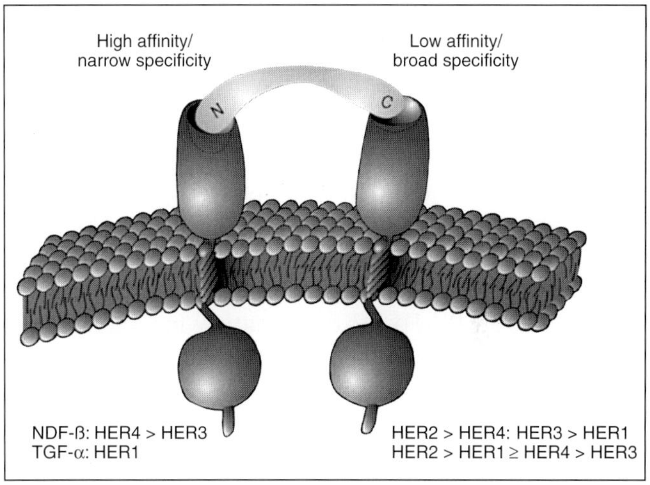

Fig. 4. Bivalence of EGF-like ligands.

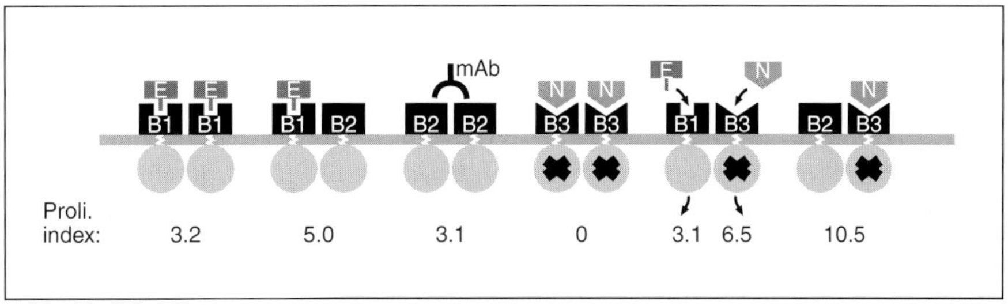

Fig. 5. The relative potency of HER dimers. Note that HER4-containing combinations were omitted. The mitogenic index of each HER dimer was calculated on the basis of experiments described in Pinkas-Kramarski et al. (Reproduced with permission from Pinkas-Kramarski et al. 1996.)

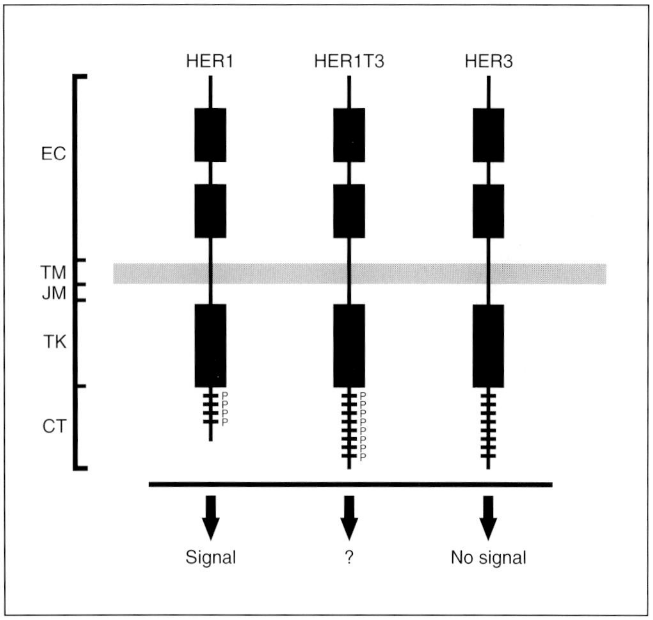

Fig. 6. HER1-HER3 chimera is the most potent receptor combination. The presented ErbB-1T3 artificial fusion protein was designed and tested in animal cells. Its activity exceeded that of the HER2-HER3 combination. (Reproduced with permission from Waterman et al. 1999.)

receptors. HER3 receptor homodimers displayed no response, even when provided with ligand. In general, HER2 heterodimers were more potent than the corresponding homodimers. Interestingly, the most active signaling complex was formed between the kinase-deficient receptor, HER3, and the ligand-less receptor, HER2. Given that the HER2-HER3 combination has the greatest mitogenic potential, we believe that this is the most relevant HER dimer to human epithelial cancer.

Heterodimers are characterized by a relatively slow rate of ligand dissociation, a feature that may explain why they generate more potent signals than homodimers [Alroy and Yarden 1997]. Heterodimers containing HER2 have a particularly high ligand binding and signaling potency compared with non-HER2 containing dimers [Karunagaren et al. 1996; Sliwkowski et al. 1994]. In addition, HER2 undergoes a slower rate of ligand-induced endocytosis compared with other HER receptors [Pinkas-Kramarski et al. 1996; Baulida et al. 1996]. Therefore, signaling by HER2 heterodimers is relatively prolonged and results in enhanced activation of signaling pathways such as the MAPK route. The relative potency of HER dimers is illustrated in figure 5. The HER2-HER3 heterodimer is the most potent mitogenic combination and is the predominant heterodimer in carcinoma cells [Alroy and Yarden 1997; Pinkas-Kramarski et al. 1998].

The HER3 receptor has only a weakly active kinase domain [Guy et al. 1994], and HER3 homodimers are mitogenically inactive [Pinkas-Kramarski et al. 1996]. However, HER3 has many docking sites for signaling molecules. It is plausible that the lack of kinase activity of HER3 prevents it from super-activating the cell. For ligand activation of HER3, it must dimerize with a HER receptor that possesses a normal kinase activity. This requirement is thought to provide increased control over the signaling activity of this rather active receptor.

In order to test this hypothesis, we engineered a chimeric HER3 receptor with kinase activity by fusing the kinase domain of HER1 to the signaling domain of HER3 [Waterman et al. 1999]. This HER1-HER3 chimera was found to be the most active receptor tested to date using this cellular system, confirming that HER3 is potentially a very active receptor. Figure 6 shows that the HER1-HER3 chimeric receptor displays greater mitogenic effect than the HER2/HER3 heterodimer and HER1 alone. This confirms that the naturally occurring HER2-HER3 dimer is the most mitogenic and suggests that the lack of kinase activity in the HER3 receptor controls the mitogenic potential of HER3. As discussed below, it is postulated that blocking the signaling activity of potent HER2-HER3 heterodimers may underlie the antiproliferative activity of HER2-targeted therapies such as Herceptin.

Signaling by Activated HER2

Considering the high level of interaction that occurs between the different HER receptors, HER signaling cannot be considered as a linear pathway. Instead, HER signaling is a very interactive system in which the ligand can lead to the formation of different homodimers or heterodimers that interact to stimulate a variety of signaling pathways. This process has been described as network signaling. The HER signal-transduction network consists of a stromal input layer (ligands or growth factors), cellular information processing layer (receptors, SH2-proteins, transcription factors), and an output layer (cell growth, differentiation or migration). Receptor dimerization is pivotal because it allows a signaling network to transmit a diverse array of biological messages. The coordination of the whole network, according to this model, is performed by HER2. Furthermore, it is believed that the absence of a HER2-specific ligand facilitates HER2-mediated regulation of the entire HER signaling network.

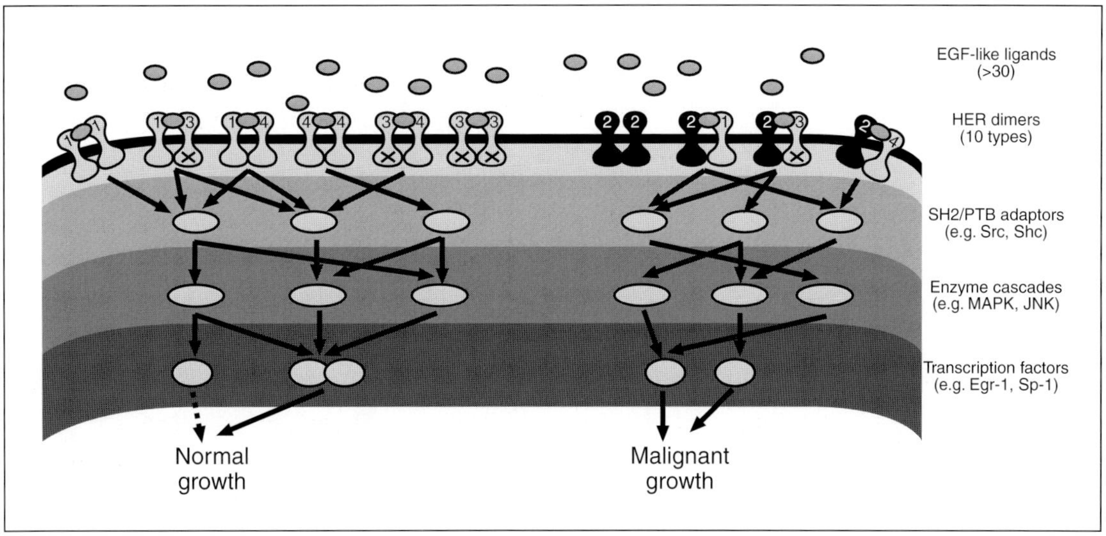

Fig. 7. The HER signaling network. The layered structure of the HER signaling network is presented. Numbers refer to the four HER proteins. Note that HER3 carries an inactive catalytic domain. (Reproduced with permission from Klapper et al. 2000.)

HER2 and Its Relevance to Cancer Immunotherapy

The HER network is illustrated in figure 7 and shows the ten different combinations of receptors in the plasma membrane. The bivalent binding to HER2-containing heterodimers allows them to bind their ligands for a longer time, which may explain the increased potency of these combinations. Other HER dimers send normal signals for cell growth and do not lead to tumor growth. The anti-HER2 monoclonal antibody (MAb), Herceptin, is thought to abolish the function of HER2, leaving only the part of the network that sends relatively weak growth signals.

Different anti-HER2 monoclonal antibodies were reported to inhibit tumor growth in mice with human tumors overexpressing a rodent oncogenic mutant of HER2 derived from human origin [Drebin et al. 1985]. We investigated the growth-inhibitory potential of a number of different antibodies to HER2 and found that the rate of tumor regression depended on the type of antibody. Whereas some antibodies almost completely abolished tumor growth, others were only partial antagonists [Stancovski et al. 1991]. Some of the anti-HER2 monoclonal antibodies were even found to enhance tumor volume. Noteworthy is that labeling of tumor cells or the antibodies revealed that tumor-promoting antibodies were not processed by the tumor cells. In contrast, the antibodies that prohibited tumor growth were rapidly internalized and metabolized by cancer cells overexpressing HER2 [Hurwitz et al. 1995]. These observations led us to propose that this results from the tumor growth inhibitory antibodies binding to HER2 on the plasma membrane, causing them to be endocytosed and moved into endocytic vesicles [Klapper et al. 2000].

Once removed from the cell surface, HER2 can no longer interact with its family members. The absence of the HER2 receptor from the signaling network prohibits the formation of potent HER2-containing heterodimers, thereby weakening growth signaling and reducing malignant growth. Consistent with this model, combining two distinct anti-HER2 antibodies produces synergistic tumor growth inhibition, probably because the combination leads to accelerated degradation of HER2 inside tumor cells [Kasprzyk et al. 1992]. These observations suggest that tumor inhibition in cancer cells overexpressing HER2 is due to the ability of HER2-specific antibodies to accelerate endocytotic removal of HER2 from the cell surface resulting in degradation of the oncoprotein.

HER2 Degradation

Research into the role of immunotherapy in enhanced endocytosis has focused on the biochemical processes leading to HER2 degradation. Generally, ligands bound

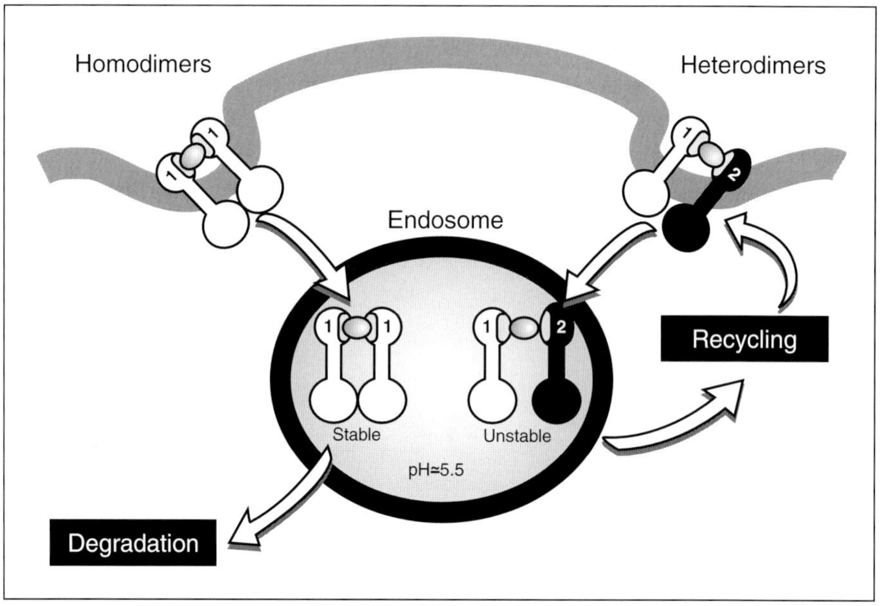

Fig. 8. HER2 promotes recycling of HER1.

to the receptor are endocytosed and these vesicles form the early endosome. In the endosome, the ligand is separated from the receptor and the receptor either recycles to the cell surface or is transported with the ligand to the lysosome, where it is degraded. The HER1 homodimer primarily goes to the lysosome and is degraded. However, when HER1 heterodimerizes with HER2, it is returned to the cell surface by HER2 (fig. 8). This recycling prolongs signaling by HER1 and probably plays a role in oncogenesis [Lenferink et al. 1998]. The sorting function that occurs in the early endosome is critical because it results in some receptors being degraded in the lysosome and some being recycled back to the cell membrane to continue signaling.

Research in this area has led to the identification of an adapter protein, c-Cbl, which controls the recycling/degradation pathway [Thien and Langdon 1998].

c-Cbl, in combination with ligand, induces degradation of receptors through the lysosome (fig. 9) [Levkowitz et al. 1998]. It appears that c-Cbl becomes associated with the receptor in the early endosome, leading to ubiquitination and subsequent degradation of the receptor in the lysosome. Unlike HER1, which strongly binds c-Cbl, HER2 only weakly interacts with this adapter molecule, and HER3 and HER4 do not recruit c-Cbl at all [Levkowitz et al. 1996]. The ring finger domain of c-Cbl, a motif that is defective in two oncogenic forms of c-Cbl, serves as a binding site for an ubiquitin-processing enzyme (E2). Coupling of c-Cbl with a specific tyrosine phosphorylated residue of HER1 enhances polyubiquitination of the receptor. Ubiquitin tags the receptor for proteosomal and lysosomal degradation [Levkowitz et al. 1999]. Interestingly, HER3, which does not carry a c-Cbl docking site, is recycled continuously [Waterman et al. 1998]. Our research with anti-HER2 antibodies suggests that antitumor antibodies tag HER2 for degradation by recruiting c-Cbl and enhancing ubiquitination of HER2. Therefore, we propose that Herceptin directs the HER2 receptor to degradation through recruitment of the c-Cbl pathway.

Thus, in this model (fig. 10), the epithelial component of the tumor responds to many mesenchymal factors from the stroma. When HER2 is overexpressed, signaling is mediated primarily by heterodimers between HER2 and other members of the HER family. These HER2 heterodimers bind the ligand quite strongly, efficiently sending signals to the nucleus to proliferate, and recycle at a high rate to the plasma membrane after endocytosis (i.e. they are long lived). This potent signaling results in increased cell multiplication and causes malignant growth. The recycling of HER2 to the plasma membrane is blocked by Herceptin-like antibodies, leading to destruction of HER2 in the lysosome. Reduced available quantities of HER2 means that the other members of the HER family cannot dimerize with HER2, so they are forced to form homodimers or heterodimers without HER2. This generates weak signaling for cell growth, thereby minimizing the potential for malignant growth.

Therapeutic Implications of HER2 Biology

HER2 protein levels in cancerous cells may be 100 times those seen in normal cells [Venter et al. 1987]. This is most commonly a consequence of gene amplification and occasionally due to transcriptional alterations. HER2 gene amplification leads to increased transcription of mRNA and synthesis of HER2 protein. In breast cancer, 92% of cases of HER2 protein overexpression are a consequence of HER2 gene amplification [Pauletti et al. 1996]. HER2 overexpression occurs in all stages of breast carcinoma and has not been identified in benign breast disease [Allred et al. 1992]. This suggests that HER2 is not amplified before the onset of true malignancy. Overexpression is maintained in metastatic lesions, suggesting a continuous function for HER2. HER2 and HER3 protein form heterodimers and co-expression of these two proteins in cells significantly increases transforming activity [Alimandi et al. 1985] predisposing to human neoplasia. This suggests that the detection of both HER2 and HER3 may have more clinical and prognostic significance than the detection of either protein alone.

Owing to the elevated levels of HER2, its accessible location at the cell surface and its role in carcinogenesis, HER2 has been under intensive scrutiny as a therapeutic target. Since HER2 is only expressed at low levels in normal tissue [De Potter et al. 1995], this allows a suitable therapeutic window to minimize damage to normal cells.

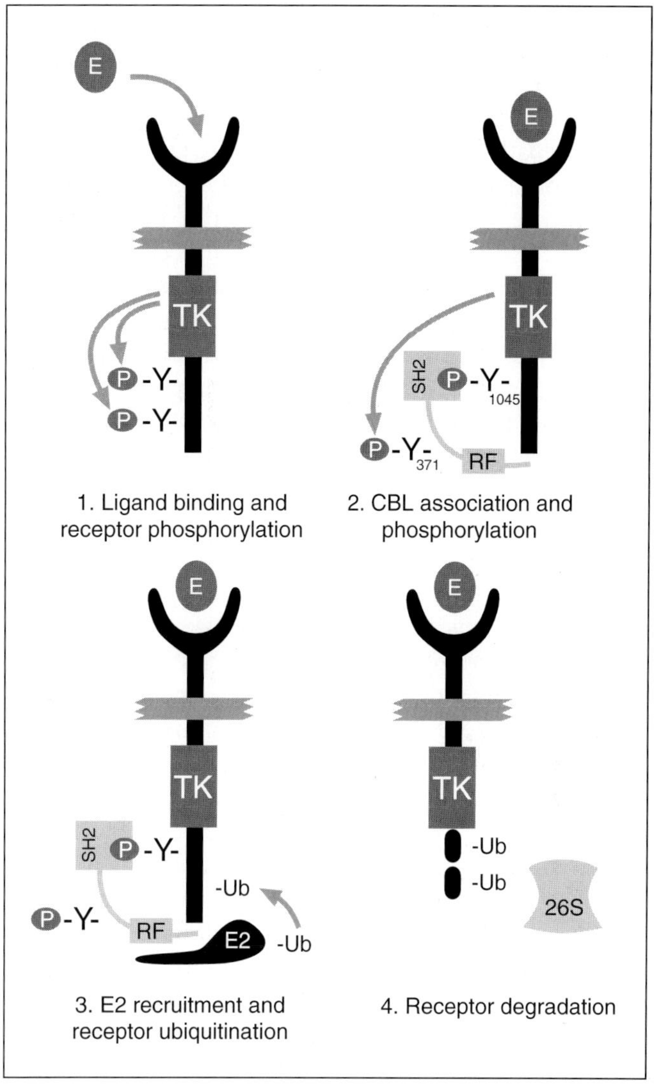

Fig. 9. Control of HER degradation.

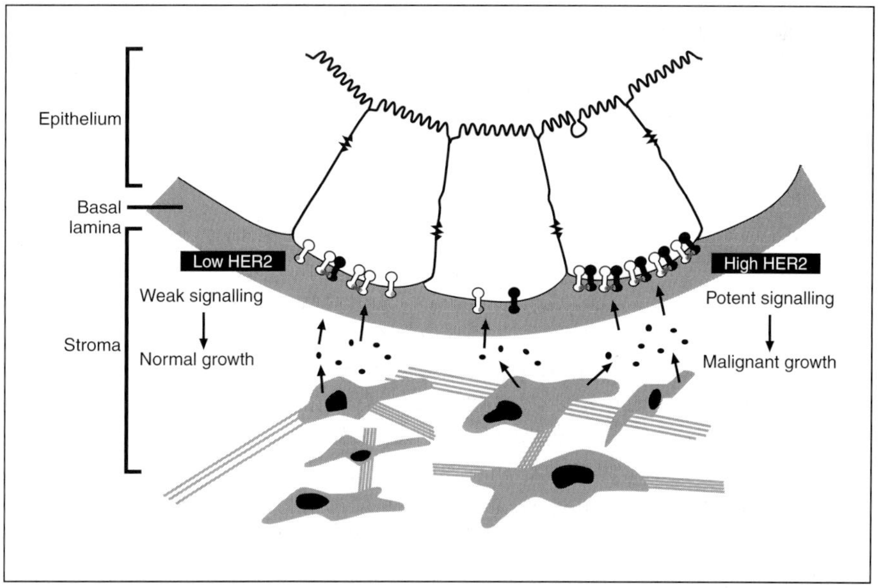

Fig. 10. HER2 controls stroma-to-epithelium crosstalk.

The HER2 protein interacts directly or indirectly with many cellular proteins, which may themselves be important in the pathogenesis of human cancer. Many of these molecules may potentially be used as targets to block the signaling pathway [Hung and Lau 1999]. However, blocking one of these proteins in the diverse signaling network may not be sufficient to totally abolish the oncogenic effect of HER2 given that other molecules can bypass the blockade. Therefore, a more effective strategy is to repress HER2 expression or to target the most upstream molecule so as to block the entire downstream signaling pathway.

The main therapeutic approaches that have been developed to target HER2-positive cancer are those that inhibit either HER2 protein function or expression [Sliwkowski et al. 1999]. One method of blocking HER2 expression involves the use of antisense constructs, either as DNA or oligonucleotides, to directly control the expression of the target gene products without affecting other cellular functions [Bertram et al. 1994; Colomer et al. 1994]. Another method of blocking the expression of HER2 is to target the HER2 promoter, e.g., by using E1A and SV40 large T antigen. An alternative strategy attempts to block the tyrosine kinase activity of the protein using a tyrosine kinase inhibitor, emodin [Hung and Lau 1999]. Another area of research involves destabilizing HER2 in the plasma membrane. For example, geldanamycin, a natural antibiotic that binds to the heat shock protein, Hsp90, is known to induce selective ubiquitination and degradation of HER receptors [Zheng et al. 2000]. Therefore, geldanamycin or analogs thereof may potentially enable the development of HER2-directed therapeutic approaches.

The most significant advances in HER2-targeted therapies have been made using MAbs directed against the extracellular domain of the HER2 protein. Several research groups have produced anti-HER2 murine MAbs (muMAbs) [Baselga and Mendelsohn 1994; Drebin et al. 1985, 1988a, b; Fendly et al. 1990; Hancock et al. 1991; Stancovski et al. 1991]. These antibodies were shown to effectively inhibit the growth of tumors and transformed cells that express high levels of HER2. The mechanism underlying their antitumor effects has not been fully elucidated although, as proposed in this paper, they may direct HER2 to the intracellular degradation pathway. However, the muMAbs did not progress beyond the experimental stages because they led to the development of human anti-mouse antibodies (HAMA). In order to circumvent the anti-globulin response during therapy a humanized MAb, rhuMAb-HER2 (trastuzumab, Herceptin), was constructed [Carter et al. 1992]. This MAb proved effective and was well tolerated in pivotal phase II and III clinical trials, both alone and in combination with chemotherapy, and has therefore been introduced into clinical practice for the treatment of patients with metastatic breast cancer [for a review see Baselga 2001].

Conclusions

The HER receptor family plays a pivotal role in the control of normal growth and differentiation. HER2 is amplified/overexpressed in a number of tumor types and is associated with reduced disease-free and overall survival in breast cancer. The exact mechanism underlying HER2 functioning and how it contributes to the virulence of human cancer has not been fully elucidated.

HER receptor proteins exist as monomers and form homo- or heterodimers on ligand binding. HER ligands are bivalent growth factor molecules. Their high-affinity site at the amino terminus has a narrow specificity and binds to HER1, HER3 or HER4, while their low-affinity site located at the carboxy terminus recruits a partner for the bound receptor. This co-receptor is typically HER2. The preference for HER2 as a co-receptor is consistent with its development as a broad-specificity receptor and the absence of a HER2-specific ligand.

HER2 exhibits a hierarchical interaction with the other HER proteins and its most potent dimerization partner is HER3, which is unique among the HER family in that it has no inherent tyrosine kinase activity. Overexpression of HER2 increases the number of HER2-HER3 heterodimers, thereby increasing HER2 signaling. HER2 heterodimers are long-lived, causing potent stroma-to-epithelium signaling and increased mitogenicity, which eventually leads to neoplastic growth. Thus, as a co-receptor and the preferred heterodimerization partner for the other HER proteins, HER2 is centrally involved in the HER signaling network and can enhance signaling by growth factors produced by tumor cells. Knocking out the signaling function of HER2 weakens growth signaling, thereby reducing malignant growth. Blocking the signaling activity of HER2-HER3 heterodimers, which are more potent than other heterodimers, may underlie the antiproliferative activity of HER2-targeted therapies such as Herceptin.

An alternative mechanism by which HER2 prolongs HER signaling is by redirecting endocytosed receptors to the recycling pathway. The sorting function that occurs in the early endosome not only reroutes HER2 to the plasma membrane to increase signaling, but also directs HER2 to lysosomal degradation sites. The process responsible for the destruction of HER2 involves recruitment of a ubiquitin ligase, c-Cbl, as well as processing by the lysosome. Removal of the HER2 receptor from the cell surface or inhibition of its intrinsic enzymatic activity may reduce oncogenicity.

HER2 is proving to be an excellent target for novel therapeutic approaches specific to HER2-overexpressing cancers such as breast cancer. Monoclonal antibodies directed against HER2, such as the humanized anti-HER2 MAb, Herceptin, represent the greatest advancement in the treatment of tumors that overexpress HER2. Our research suggests that the antitumor efficacy of HER2-specific MAbs such as Herceptin may relate to their ability to direct HER2 to a Cbl-dependent endocytosis and degradation pathway. The reported clinical therapeutic efficacy of anti-HER2 MAbs in breast cancer highlights the importance of understanding the biology of HER2. Further elucidation of the role of HER2 in cell growth will help to develop additional innovative therapies for the management of patients with HER2-positive disease.

References

Akiyama T, Saito T, Ogawara H, Toyoshima K, Yamamoto T: Tumor promoter and epidermal growth factor stimulate phosphorylation of the c-erbB-2 gene product in MKN-7 human adenocarcinoma cells. Mol Cell Biol 1988;8:1019–1026.

Akiyama T, Sudo C, Ogawara H, Toyoshima K, Yamamoto T: The product of the human c-erbB-2 gene: A 185-kilodalton glycoprotein with tyrosine kinase activity. Science 1986; 232:1644–1646.

Alimandi M, Romano A, Curia MC, Muraro R, Fedi P, Aaronson SA, Di Fiore PP, Kraus MH: Cooperative signaling of erbB3 and erbB2 in neoplastic transformation and human mammary carcinomas. Oncogene 1985;10:1813–1821.

Allred DC, Clarke GM, Molina R, Tandon AK, Schnitt SJ, Gilchrist KW, Osborne CK, Tormey DC, McGuire WL: Overexpression of HER-2/*neu* and its relationship with other prognostic factors change during the progression of in situ to invasive breast cancer. Hum Pathol 1992;23:974–979.

Alroy I, Yarden Y: The ErbB signaling network in embryogenesis and oncogenesis: signal diversification through combinatorial ligand-receptor interactions. FEBS Lett 1997;410:83–86.

American Society of Clinical Oncology (ASCO): 1997 update of recommendations for the use of tumour markers in breast and colorectal cancer. J Clin Oncol 1998;16:793–795.

Baly DL, Wirth CM, Allison DA et al: Development and characterization of a rhuMAb HER2 antibody assay for clinical evaluation of cytotoxic potency. Proc Am Assoc Cancer Res 1997;38:181A.

Bargmann CI, Hung MC, Weinberg RA: The neu oncogene encodes an epidermal growth factor receptor-related protein. Nature 1986;319: 226–230.

Baselga J: Herceptin® alone or in combination with chemotherapy in the treatment of HER2-positive metastatic breast cancer: pivotal trials. Oncology 2001;61(suppl 2):14–21.

Baselga J, Mendelsohn J: Receptor blockade with monoclonal antibodies as anticancer therapy. Pharmacol Ther 1994;64:127–154.

Baulida J, Kraus MH, Alimandi M, Di Fiore PP, Carpenter G: All ErbB receptors other than the epidermal growth factor receptor are endocytosis impaired. J Biol Chem 1996;271:5251–5257.

Berchuck A, Kamel A, Whitaker R, Kerns B, Olt G, Kinney R, Soper JT, Dodge R, Clarke-Pearson DL, Marks P, et al: Overexpression of HER-2/neu is associated with poor survival in advanced epithelial ovarian cancer. Cancer Res 1990;50:4087–4091.

Bertram J, Killian M, Brysch W, Schlingensiepen KH, Kneba M: Reduction of erbB2 gene product in mammary carcinoma cell lines by erbB2 mRNA specific and tyrosine kinase consensus phosphorothioate antisense oligonucleotides. Biochem Biophys Res Commun 1994;200: 661–667.

Burden S, Yarden Y: Neuregulins and their receptors: a versatile signaling module in organogenesis and oncogenesis. Neuron 1997;18:847–855.

Carraway KL 3rd, Weber JL, Unger MJ, Ledesma J, Yu N, Gassmann M, Lai C: Neuregulin-2, a new ligand of erbB3/erbB4-receptor tyrosine kinases. Nature 1997;387:512–516.

Carter P, Presta L, Gorman CM, Ridgway JB, Henner D, Wong WL, Rowland AM, Kotts C, Carver ME, Shepard HM: Humanization of the anti-p185HER2 antibody for human cancer therapy. Proc Natl Acad Sci USA 1992;89: 4285–4289.

Colomer R, Lupu R, Bacus SS, Gelmann EP: erbB-2 antisense oligonucleotides inhibit the proliferation of breast carcinoma cells with erbB-2 oncogene amplification. Br J Cancer 1994;70: 819–825.

Cooke T: What is HER2? Eur J Oncology Nursing 2000;4(suppl 1):2–9.

Connelly PA, Stern DF: The epidermal growth factor receptor and the product of the neu-protooncogene are members of a receptor tyrosine phosphorylation cascade. Proc Natl Acad Sci USA 1990:87:6054–6057.

Coussens L, Yang-Fen TL, Liao Y-C, Chen E, Gray A, McGrath J, Seeburg PH, Libermann TA, Schlessinger J, Francke U, Levinson A, Ullrich A: Tyrosine kinase receptor with extensive homology to EGF receptor shares chromosomal location with *neu* oncogene. Science 1985;230: 1132–1139.

De Potter CR, Schelfhout AM, Verbeek P, Lakhani SR, Brunken R, Schroeter CA, Van den Tweel JG, Schauer AJ, Sloane JP: Neu overexpression correlates with extent of disease in large cell ductal in situ carcinoma of the breast. Hum Pathol 1995;26:601–606.

Devesa SS, Blot WJ, Stone BJ, Miller BA, Tarone RE, Fraumeni JF Jr: Recent cancer trends in the United States. J Natl Cancer Inst 1995;87: 175–182.

Di Augustine R, Richards RG: EGF-related peptides and their receptors in mammary gland development. Journal of Mammary Gland Biology and Neoplasia 1997;2:109–118.

Drebin JA, Link VC, Stern DF, Weinberg RA, Greene MI: Down-modulation of an oncogene protein product and reversion of the transformed phenotype by monoclonal antibodies. Cell 1985;41:697–706.

Drebin JA, Link VC, Greene MI: Monoclonal antibodies reactive with distinct domains of the neu oncogene-encoded p185 molecule exert synergistic anti-tumor effects in vivo. Oncogene 1988a;2:273–277.

Drebin JA, Link VC, Greene MI: Monoclonal antibodies specific for the neu oncogene product directly mediate anti-tumor effects in vivo. Oncogene 1988b;2:387–394.

Estéve J, Kricker A, Ferlay J, Parkin DM in collaboration with the Steering Committee of the European Network of Cancer Registries; in Facts and Figures of Cancer in the European Community. Paris, International Agency for Research on Cancer, 1996.

Fendly BM, Winget M, Hudziak RM, Lipari MT, Napier MA, Ullrich A: Characterization of murine monoclonal antibodies reactive to either the human growth factor receptor or HER2/*neu* gene product. Cancer Res 1990;50:1550–1558.

Guy PM, Platko JV, Cantley LC, Cerione RA, Carraway KL: Insect cell-expressed p180ErbB3 possesses an impaired tyrosine kinase activity. Proc Natl Acad Sci USA 1994;91:8132–8136.

Hancock MC, Langton BC, Chan T, Toy P, Monahan JJ, Mischak RP, Shawver LK: A monoclonal antibody against the c-erbB-2 protein enhances the cytotoxicity of cis-diaminedichloroplatinum against human breast and ovarian tumor cell lines. Cancer Res 1991;51: 4575–4580.

Hou L, Shi D, Tu SM, Zhang HZ, Hung MC, Ling D: Oral cancer progression and c-erbB-2/neu proto-oncogene expression. Cancer Lett 1992; 65:215–220.

Hung MC, Lau Y-K: Basic science of HER2/neu: a review. Semin Oncol 1999;26:51–59.

Hung MC, Schechter AL, Chevray PY, Stem DF, Weinberg RA: Molecular cloning of the neu gene: Absence of gross structural alteration in oncogenic alleles. Proc Natl Acad Sci USA 1986;83:261–264.

Hurwitz E, Stancovski I, Sela M, Yarden Y: Suppression and promotion of tumor growth by monoclonal antibodies to ErbB-2 differentially correlate with cellular uptake. Proc Natl Acad Sci USA 1995;92:3353–3357.

Hynes NE, Stern DF: The biology of *erb*B-2/*neu*/*HER*-2 and its role in cancer. Biochim Biophys Acta Rev Cancer 1994;1198:165–184.

Jones FE, Jerry DJ, Guarino BC, Andrews GC, Stem DF: Heregulin induced in vivo proliferation and differentiation of mammary epithelium into secretory lobuloalveoli. Cell Growth Differ 1996;7:1031–1038.

Karunagaren D, Tzahar E, Beerli RR, Chen X, Graus-Porta D, Ratzkin BJ, Seger R, Hynes NE, Yarden Y: ErbB-2 is a common auxiliary subunit of NDF and EGF receptors: implications for breast cancer. EMBO J 1996;15:254–264.

Kasprzyk PG, Song SU, Di Fiore PP, King CR: Therapy of an animal model of human gastric cancer using a combination of anti-erbB-2 monoclonal antibodies. Cancer Res 1992;52:2771–2776.

Klapper LN, Kirschbaum MH, Sela M, Yarden Y: Biochemical and clinical implications of the ErbB/HER signaling network of growth factor receptors; in Klein G, Woude V (eds): Advances in Cancer Research. Academic Press, 2000, pp 25–79.

Klapper LN, Glathe S, Vaisman N, Hynes NE, Andrews GC, Sela M, Yarden Y: The ErbB-2/HER2 oncoprotein of human carcinomas may function solely as a shared coreceptor for multiple stroma-derived growth factors. Proc Natl Acad Sci USA 1999;96:4995–5000.

Kokai Y, Meyers JN, Wada T, Brown VI, LeVea CM, Davis JG, Dobashi K, Greene MI: Synergistic interaction of p185c-neu and the EGF receptor leads to transformation of rodent fibroblasts. Cell 1989;58:287–292.

Lenferink AE, Pinkas-Kramarski R, Van de Poll ML, Klapper LN, Tzahar E, Waterman H, Sela M, Van-Zoelen EY, Yarden Y: Differential endocytic routing of homo- and hetero-dimeric ErbB tyrosine kinases confers signaling superiority to receptor heterodimers. EMBO J 1998; 17:3385–3397.

Levkowitz G, Klapper LN, Tzahar E, Freywald A, Sela M, Yarden Y: Coupling of the c-Cbl protooncogene product to ErbB-1/EGF-receptor but not to other ErbB proteins. Oncogene 1996;12: 1117–1125.

Levkowitz G, Waterman H, Ettenberg SA, Katz M, Tsygankov AY, Alroy I, Lavi S, Iwai K, Reiss Y, Ciechenover A, Lipkowitz S, Yarden Y: Ubiquitin ligase activity and tyrosine phosphorylation underlie suppression of growth factor signaling by c-Cbl/Sli-1. Mol Cell 1999;4: 1029–1040.

Levkowitz G, Waterman H, Zamir L, Kam Z, Oved S, Langdon WY, Beguinot L, Geiger B, Yarden Y: c-Cbl/Sli-1 regulates endocytic sorting and ubiquitination of the epidermal growth factor receptor. Genes Dev 1998;12:3663–3674.

Lupu R, Cardillo M, Harris L, Hijazi M, Rosenberg K: Interaction between ERB-receptors and heregulin in breast cancer tumor progression and drug resistance. Sem Cancer Biol 1995:6:135–145.

McCann AH, Dervan PA, O'Regan M, Codd MB, Gullick WJ, Tobin BM, Carney DN: Prognostic significance of c-erbB-2 and estrogen receptor status in human breast cancer. Cancer Res 1991;51:3296–3303.

Meyer C, Birchmeier C: Multiple essential functions of neuregulin in development. Nature 1995;378:386–390.

Normanno N, Ciardiello F: EGF-related peptides in the pathophysiology of the mammary gland. J Mammary Gland Biol Neoplasia 1997;2: 143–152.

Pauletti G, Godolphin W, Press MF, Slamon DJ: Detection and quantitation of HER-2/neu gene amplification in human breast cancer archival material using fluorescence in situ hybridization. Oncogene 1996;13:63–72.

Piccart M, Lohrisch C, Di Leo A, Larsimont D: The predictive value of HER2 in breast cancer. Oncology 2001;61(suppl 2):73–82.

Pinkas-Kramarski R, Eilam R, Alroy I, Levkowitz G, Lonai P, Yarden Y: Differential expression of NDF/neuregulin receptors ErbB-3 and ErbB-4 and involvement in inhibition of neuronal differentiation. Oncogene 1997;15:803–815.

Pinkas-Kramarski R, Shelly M, Guarino BC, Wang LM, Lyass L, Alroy I, Alimandi M, Kuo A, Moyer JD, Lavi S, Eisenstein M, Ratzkin BJ, Seger R, Bacus SS, Pierce JH, Andrews GC, Yarden Y, Alamandi M: ErbB tyrosine kinases and the two neuregulin families constitute a ligand-receptor network. Mol Cell Biol 1998; 18:6090–6101.

Pinkas-Kramarski R, Soussan L, Waterman H, Levkowitz G, Alroy I, Klapper L, Lavi S, Seger R, Ratzkin BJ, Sela M, Yarden Y: Diversification of Neu differentiation factor and epidermal growth factor signaling by combinatorial receptor interactions. EMBO J 1996;15:2452–2467.

Quirke P, Pickles A, Tuzi NL, Mohamdee O, Gullick WJ: Pattern of expression of c-erbB-2 oncoprotein in human fetuses. Br J Cancer 1989; 60:64–69.

Ross JS, Fletcher JA: The Her-2/neu oncogene in breast cancer: prognostic factor, predictive factor, and target for therapy. Stem Cells 1998;16: 413–428.

Schneider PM, Hung MC, Chiocco SM, Manning J, Zhao XY, Fung K, Roth JA: Differential expression of the c-erbB-2 gene in human small cell and non-small cell lung cancer. Cancer Res 1989;49:4968–4971.

Slamon DJ, Clark GM, Wong SG, Levin WJ, Ullrich A, McGuire WL: Human breast cancer: correlation of relapse and survival with amplification of the HER-2/neu oncogene. Science 1987;235:177–182.

Slamon DJ, Godolphin W, Jones LA, Holt JA, Wong SG, Keith DE, Levin WJ, Stuart SG, Udove J, Ullrich A, et al: Studies of the HER2/neu proto-oncogene in human and breast ovarian cancer. Science 1989;244:707–712.

Sliwkowski MX, Schaefer G, Akita RW, Lofgren JA, Fitzpatrick VD, Nuijens A, Fendly BM, Cerione RA, Vandlen RL, Carraway KL: Coexpression of erbB2 and erbB3 proteins reconstitutes a high affinity receptor for heregulin. J Biol Chem 1994;269:14661–14665.

Sliwkowski MX, Lofgren JA, Lewis GD, Hotaling TE, Fendly BM, Fox JA: Nonclinical studies addressing the mechanism of action of trastuzumab (Herceptin). Semin Oncol 1999;26:60–70.

Stancovski I, Hurwitz E, Leitner O, Ullrich A, Yarden Y, Sela M: Mechanistic aspects of the opposing effects of monoclonal antibodies to the ERBB2 receptor on tumor growth. Proc Natl Acad Sci USA 1991;88:8691–8695.

Thien CBF, Langdon W: c-Cbl: a regulator of T cell receptor-mediated signaling. Immunol Cell Biol 1998;76:473–82.

Tzahar E, Pinkas-Kramarski R, Moyer JD, Klapper LN, Alroy I, Levkowitz G, Shelly M, Henis S, Eisenstein M, Ratzkin BJ, Sela M, Andrews GC, Yarden Y: Bivalence of EGF-like ligands drives the ErbB signaling network. EMBO J 1997;16:4938–4950.

Tzahar E, Waterman H, Chen X, Levkowitz G, Karunagaran D, Lavi S, Ratzkin BJ, Yarden Y: A hierarchical network of interreceptor interactions determines signal transduction by Neu differentiation factor/neuregulin and epidermal growth factor. Mol Cell Biol 1996;16: 5276–5287.

Tzahar E, Yarden Y: The ErbB-2/HER2 oncogenic receptor of adenocarcinomas: from orphanhood to multiple stromal ligands. BBA Rev Cancer 1998;1377:25–37.

van de Vijver M, van de Bersselaar R, Devilee P, Cornelisse C, Peterse J, Nusse R: Amplification of the neu/c-erbB-2 oncogene in human mammary tumors is relatively frequent and is often accompanied by amplification of the linked c-erbA oncogene. Mol Cell Biol 1987;7:2019–2023.

van der Geer P, Hunter T, Lindberg RA: Receptor protein-tyrosine kinases and their signal transduction pathways. Annu Rev Cell Biol 1994; 10:251–337.

Vennstrom B, Bishop JM: Isolation and characterization of chicken DNA homologous to the two putative oncogenes of avian erythroblastosis virus. Cell 1982;28:135–143.

Venter DJ, Tuzi NL, Kumar S, Gullick WJ: Overexpression of the c-erbB-2 oncoprotein in human breast carcinomas: immunohistological assessment correlates with gene amplification. Lancet 1987;ii:69–72.

Waterman H, Alroy I, Strano S, Seger R, Yarden Y: The carboxyl terminus of the kinase-defective neuregulin receptor ErbB-3 confers mitogenic superiority and dictates endocytic routing. EMBO J 1999;18:3348–3358.

Waterman H, Sabanai I, Geiger B, Yarden Y: Alternative intracellular routing of ErbB receptors may determine signaling potency. J Biol Chem 1998;273:13819–13827.

Weiner DB, Nordberg J, Robinson R, Nowell PC, Gazdar A, Greene MI, Williams WV, Cohen JA, Kern JA: Expression of the neu gene-encoded protein (P185neu) in human non-small cell carcinomas of the lung. Cancer Res 1990;50:421–425.

Xia W, Lau Y-K, Zhang H-Z, Liu AR, Li L, Kiyokawa N, Clayman GL, Katz RL, Hung MC: Strong correlation between c-erbB-2 overexpression and overall survival of patients with oral squamous cell carcinoma. Clin Cancer Res 1997;3:3–9.

Yamamoto T, Ikawa S, Akiyama T, Semba K, Nomura N, Miyajima N, Saito T, Toyoshima K: Similarity of protein encoded by the human c-erb-2 gene to epidermal growth factor receptor. Nature 1986;319:230–234.

Yang T, Spitzer E, Meyer D, Sachs M, Niemann C, Hartman G, Weidner KM, Birchmeier C, Birchmeier W: Sequential requirement of hepatocyte growth factor and neuregulin in the morphogenesis and differentiation of the mammary gland. J Cell Biol 1995;131:215–226.

Yokota J, Yamamoto T, Miyajima N, Toyoshima K, Nomura N, Sakamoto H, Yoshida T, Terada M, Sugimura T: Genetic alterations of the c-erbB-2 oncogene occur frequently in tubular adenocarcinoma of the stomach and are often accompanied by amplification of the v-erbA homologue. Oncogene 1988;2:283–287.

Yoshida K, Tsuda T, Matsumura T, Tsujino T, Hattori T, Ito H, Tahara E: Amplification of epidermal growth factor receptor (EGFR) gene and oncogenes in human gastric carcinomas. Virchows Arch B Cell Pathol Mol Pathol 1989; 57:285–290.

Zhang X, Silva E, Gersenhson D, Hung MC: Amplification and re-arrangement of c-erbB protooncogenes in cancer of human female genital tract. Oncogene 1989;4:985–989.

Zheng EF, Kuduk SD, Chiosis G, Munster PN, Sepp-Lorenzino L, Danishefsky SJ, Rosen N: Identification of a geldanamycin dimer that induces selective degradation of HER-family tyrosine kinases. Cancer Res 2000;60:2090–2094.

Oncology

Oncology 2001;61(suppl 2):14–21

Herceptin® Alone or in Combination with Chemotherapy in the Treatment of HER2-Positive Metastatic Breast Cancer: Pivotal Trials

José Baselga

Medical Oncology Service, Hospital General, Universitari Vall d'Hebron, Barcelona, Spain

Key Words

FISH · HER2 positive · Herceptin® · IHC 3+ · Metastatic breast cancer · Pivotal trial · Survival benefit

Abstract

Large pivotal phase II and III clinical trials investigated the therapeutic efficacy and safety of the humanized anti-HER2 monoclonal antibody, Herceptin®, alone and in combination with standard chemotherapy, respectively, in HER2-positive metastatic breast cancer. Eligible patients were HER2 2+ and 3+ overexpressors, as determined by immunohistochemistry (IHC). Herceptin was well tolerated in both trials. Single-agent second/third-line Herceptin produced durable tumor responses. First-line Herceptin in combination with chemotherapy, in particular paclitaxel, significantly improved time to disease progression, duration of response and time to treatment failure. Combination therapy also provided a significant 25% improvement in overall survival. These clinical benefits have led to the approval of Herceptin for clinical use in the USA and elsewhere. Greater efficacy was noted in IHC 3+ patients compared with the overall population in both trials. Retrospective fluorescent in situ hybridization (FISH) testing of patient-tumor HER2 status revealed similar clinical outcomes in IHC 3+ and FISH-positive patients, consistent with the reported high concordance between IHC and FISH. Responses in the single-agent Herceptin trial were seen exclusively in FISH-positive patients. Approximately a quarter of HER2 2+ patients test FISH positive and may therefore benefit from therapy. Numerous studies are underway or planned to evaluate other Herceptin combinations and regimens in the metastatic and adjuvant settings.

Introduction

The human epidermal growth factor receptor-2 (HER2) is a growth factor receptor protein encoded by the HER2 oncogene [Coussens et al. 1985; Hynes and Stern 1994]. The HER2 gene is also known as HER2/*neu* or c-*erb*B2 and encodes a 185-kD transmembrane glycoprotein receptor ($p185^{HER2}$). HER2 belongs to a family of genes involved in the regulation of normal breast growth and development. HER2 overexpression is detected in many types of tumor [Hynes and Stern 1994] and is known to be associated with the pathogenesis of breast cancer. HER2 receptor overexpression is almost exclusively the result of amplification of the HER2 gene, which leads to the oncogenic transformation of normal cells [Di Fiore et al. 1987a, b; Hudziak et al. 1987].

KARGER

Fax + 41 61 306 12 34
E-Mail karger@karger.ch
www.karger.com

0030–2414/01/0616–0014$17.50/0

Accessible online at:
www.karger.com/journals/ocl

J. Baselga, MD
Hospital Vall d'Hebron, Department of Medical Oncology
Pg. Vall d'Hebron, 119–129
E–08035 Barcelona (Spain)
Tel. +34 93 274 6077, Fax +34 93 274 6059, E-Mail baselga@hg.vhebron.es

HER2 amplification/overexpression correlates with poor clinical outcome in both node-positive and node-negative patients, with these patients having more aggressive disease and a shortened overall survival when compared with patients with HER2-negative tumors [Hynes and Stern 1994; Ravdin et al. 1995; Slamon et al. 1987, 1989]. Furthermore, preclinical data suggest that HER2 overexpression is not just a marker of tumor status, but that it actually contributes directly to the tumor phenotype [Di Fiore et al. 1987b; Guy et al. 1992; Ménard 2001; Hudziak et al. 1987]. Targeted therapeutic agents directed against either HER2 overexpression or the function of the HER2 protein have been developed with a view to improving clinical benefit and tolerability compared with traditional cytotoxic approaches.

Preclinical studies have demonstrated that anti-HER2 monoclonal antibodies (MAb) can inhibit the growth of HER2-overexpressing tumor cells [Hancock et al. 1991; Hudziak et al. 1989; McKenzie et al. 1989; Stancovski et al. 1991]. In particular, the humanized anti-HER2 MAb, Herceptin® (trastuzumab), has been shown to promote enhanced antiproliferative/antitumor effects in HER2-overexpressing breast cancer cell lines and tumor xenograft models [Baselga et al. 1998; Carter et al. 1992; Lewis et al. 1993]. Early clinical trials using recombinant Herceptin have demonstrated the efficacy of this targeted approach in the treatment of HER2-positive breast cancer patients who have relapsed following conventional treatment for their metastatic disease [Baselga et al. 1996; Pegram et al. 1998]. This paper reports on the results of two pivotal Herceptin trials: a phase II trial of second-/third-line single-agent Herceptin [Cobleigh et al. 1999]; and a phase III combination trial comparing Herceptin plus chemotherapy versus chemotherapy alone as first-line treatment for patients with HER2-positive metastatic breast cancer [Mass et al. 2000; Norton et al. 1999; Slamon et al. 1998, 2001]. The efficacy data are reported for both trials and discussed in relation to levels of HER2 amplification/overexpression as measured by fluorescence in situ hybridization (FISH) and immunohistochemistry (IHC), respectively.

Determination of HER2 Status

For both pivotal trials, HER2-positive patients were identified using an IHC-based assay termed the clinical trials assay (CTA). This was performed using either 4D5 or CB11 anti-HER2 antibodies. Patients were eligible for enrollment if their HER2 overexpression scored IHC 2+ or 3+ on at least one of the assays. If both assays were employed, the higher of the two results was used.

An alternative to IHC for determining HER2 status is FISH. This method measures the level of HER2 gene amplification. The PathVysion™ kit (Vysis) has been approved by the FDA as an adjunct to existing clinical and pathological information. The kit contains two probes, a HER2-specific probe and a chromosome 17 centromeric probe that is used as a control. Nuclei from 60 cells are enumerated and the ratio of the HER2 signal to the chromosome 17 signal determined. Tumors are graded FISH positive if the HER2:chromosome 17 ratio for amplification is two or greater.

Table 1. Concordance between IHC and FISH performed according to the clinical trials assay on patient tissues from the pivotal trials

	0	1+	2+	3+
FISH–	207	28	67	21
FISH+	7 (3%)	2 (7%)	21 (24%)	176 (89%)

Overall concordance = 82%.

IHC/FISH Concordance Data

Retrospective analysis of patient tissue samples from the pivotal Herceptin trials by FISH (PathVysion™) allowed the concordance between the CTA and FISH to be determined. The overall concordance between the CTA and FISH was 82% [Mass et al. 2000]. Moreover, concordance between IHC 3+ and FISH-positive tumors was even greater (89%). In contrast, concordance between IHC 2+ tumors and FISH positivity was 24% (table 1).

Pivotal Phase II Single-Agent Trial

Study Design

All patients included in the pivotal, phase II, multicenter, open-label, single-arm Herceptin trial had progressive disease after one or two cytotoxic chemotherapy regimens for metastatic disease [Cobleigh et al. 1999]. The trial was conducted to determine response rate as defined by complete and partial responses (CR and PR, respectively). Response rates were assessed by a blinded, independent Response Evaluation Committee (REC) at weeks 8, 16, 24 and every 12 weeks thereafter. Secondary endpoints in this trial were duration of response (DR), time to disease progression (TTP), time to treatment failure (TTF) and survival. Adverse events and health-related quality of life (QoL) were also measured: QoL was assessed using the EORTC core QoL questionnaire (QLQ-C30). The median follow-up for all patients was 12.8 months: the final analyses of efficacy and safety were performed 15 months after the last patient was enrolled.

Treatment

A total of 222 patients from 54 centers were enrolled into the phase II trial. Herceptin was administered as a 4-mg/kg intravenous loading dose followed by a weekly intravenous infusion of 2 mg/kg. If a patient developed progressive disease the investigator could continue the 2-mg/kg dose, increase it to 4 mg/kg weekly or discontinue treatment. Additional antitumor therapy was permitted upon disease progression. Two hundred thirteen patients received at least one dose of Herceptin. Nine patients were not treated for the following reasons: brain metastases (n = 3), laboratory abnormality (n = 2), adverse event (n = 1), refusal to participate (n = 1), clinical instability (n = 1) and death (n = 1).

Efficacy

The REC documented eight complete (4%) and 26 partial (11%) responses to yield an overall objective response rate (ORR) of 15% in the intent to treat (ITT) patient population. In addition, there were 12 minor responses (6%) and 62 patients (29%) with stable disease (SD). The median DR in Herceptin-treated patients was 9.1 months (range 1.6 to >26 months).

The investigator-assessed response rate was 22% [Cobleigh et al. 1999]. In addition to the patients who achieved a response, the investigators identified a subset of patients who experienced SD for longer than 6 months. Adding the responders to those patients with SD >6 months provides an overall clinical benefit of 30%.

Eight (24%) of the 34 responding patients were free of disease progression at the cut-off date. After a median follow-up of 12.8 months, the median TTP was 3.1 months (range 0 to >28 months) and the median TTF was 2.4 months (range 0 to >28 months) for all treated patients. The median TTF among the 34 responding patients was 11 months (range 2 to >28 months). This contrasted with a median TTF of 5.4 months (range 0 to >27.4 months) for the same patients on their prior cytotoxic chemotherapy regimens. Median survival for all patients was 13 months (range 0.5 to >30 months). A total of 154 patients completed the QLQ-C30 questionnaire. The results indicated that Herceptin improved global QoL and social function over baseline [Lieberman et al. 1999].

Subgroup Analyses

Correlation of tumor response with level of HER2 overexpression showed that IHC 3+ patients had a better response rate than the overall (IHC 2+ and 3+) patient population (18 vs. 15%, respectively) [Cobleigh et al. 1999]. Similarly, IHC 3+ patients demonstrated a longer median duration of survival than the overall population (16.4 versus 13 months).

Sixty percent of samples from the pivotal Herceptin trials were retested using FISH. This allowed a retrospective analysis of tumor response based on FISH status. In the pivotal phase II Herceptin single-agent trial, the response rate was 20% in FISH-positive patients and 0% in FISH-negative patients [Mass et al. 2000]. All patients in the IHC 2+ and 3+ subgroups who responded tested FISH positive. These results suggest that FISH assessment of HER2 gene amplification may allow the selection of all HER2-positive patients who will benefit from Herceptin therapy.

Safety

The safety of Herceptin therapy is reviewed in detail elsewhere [Cook-Bruns 2001]. In brief, Herceptin was generally well tolerated as a single-agent in the pivotal phase II trial. As with other antibody therapies, infusion-related fever and/or chills were reported during the first Herceptin administration, occurring in about 40% of patients. All other side effects were minor with the exception of cardiac dysfunction, which was determined to occur in 10 patients. However, nine of the 10 patients were considered to have pre-existing conditions that would predispose to this adverse event. Of particular note, adverse events typically associated with cytotoxic agents were not demonstrated with Herceptin therapy.

Pivotal Phase III Combination Trial

Study Design

The pivotal, randomized, multicenter, phase III Herceptin combination trial was conducted to evaluate both the clinical efficacy and safety of Herceptin used in combination with chemotherapy versus chemotherapy alone [Mass et al. 2000; Norton et al. 1999; Slamon et al. 1998, 2001]. Patients eligible for entry into the trial had HER2-positive metastatic breast cancer but had not received prior therapy for metastatic disease.

Table 2. Efficacy of Herceptin given in combination with chemotherapy in all patients and IHC 3+ patients

	H+AC (n = 143)	AC (n = 138)	H+P (n = 92)	P (n = 96)	H+CT (n = 235)	CT (n = 234)
Median TTP, months						
All	7.8*	6.1	6.9*	2.7	7.4*	4.6
3+	8.1*	6.0	7.1*	3.0	7.8*	4.6
RR, %	56	42	41	17	50	32
	60	42	49	17	56	31
Median DR, months	9.1	6.7	10.5	4.5	9.1	6.1
	9.3	5.9	10.9	4.6	10.0	5.6
Median TTF, months	7.0*	5.6	5.3*	2.7	6.6*	4.5
	7.1	5.1	6.7	2.8	7.0	4.4
Survival, months	27	21	22	18	25*	20
	31*	21	25	18	29*	20

* $p < 0.05$. All: n = 469; 3+: n = 349.

The primary study endpoints of the study were TTP and the safety of Herceptin when used as first-line therapy concomitantly with other anticancer agents. Secondary endpoints were overall response rate (ORR), duration of response (DR), time to treatment failure (TTF), one-year survival and QoL. Tumor responses were assessed by an independent REC at weeks 8 and 20 and at 12-weekly intervals thereafter. The median follow-up was 35 months (cut-off October 1999).

Treatment

Four hundred sixty-nine patients were randomized to receive either chemotherapy alone (n = 234) or Herceptin plus chemotherapy (n = 235). The type of chemotherapy received in this trial depended on which therapies had previously been given for adjuvant disease. If patients had not had prior adjuvant anthracycline therapy, they were randomized to receive anthracycline (either doxorubicin 60 mg/m^2 or epirubicin 75 mg/m^2) plus cyclophosphamide 600 mg/m^2 (AC) alone (n = 138) or in combination with Herceptin (n = 143). Patients who had received prior anthracycline therapy in an adjuvant setting were randomized to receive paclitaxel (175 mg/m^2) alone (n = 96) or in combination with Herceptin (n = 92) (table 1).

Herceptin was administered as described previously (4 mg/kg initial dose followed by weekly 2 mg/kg intravenous infusions) until disease progression. AC was given intravenously every 3 weeks over a minimum of 6 cycles. Paclitaxel was administered as a 3-hour intravenous infusion every 3 weeks over a minimum of 6 cycles. Following disease progression, patients randomized to receive chemotherapy alone could cross over to an extension study to receive Herceptin therapy.

Time to Disease Progression

After a median follow-up of 35 months, addition of Herceptin to chemotherapy was associated with a significantly improved TTP of 7.4 months compared with 4.6 months for those patients receiving chemotherapy alone ($p < 0.05$; table 2). Significantly, the increase in TTP was greater in the Herceptin plus paclitaxel subgroup (6.9 versus 2.7 months; $p < 0.05$) than in the Herceptin plus AC subgroup (7.8 versus 6.1 months; $p < 0.05$).

Tumor Response Rates

Patients receiving Herceptin combination therapy had a greater ORR (50%) than those receiving chemotherapy alone (32%). A longer median DR of 9.1 months was also associated with the combination therapy; the median DR for chemotherapy alone was 6.1 months. Herceptin combination therapy also prolonged the median TTF (table 2). In addition, improvements were noted in the individual Herceptin plus chemotherapy subgroups. The addition of Herceptin to paclitaxel significantly improved the RR from 17 to 41% ($p < 0.0001$), and the median DR from 4.5 to 10.5 months ($p < 0.001$) compared with paclitaxel therapy alone (table 2). Similarly, the addition of Herceptin to AC improved the RR from 42 to 56% and the median DR from 6.7 to 9.1 months compared with AC therapy alone.

Median Survival

In the phase III trial, Herceptin combination therapy was associated with a significantly improved median survival (25 months) compared with that observed following chemotherapy alone (20 months; $p < 0.05$). This enhancement of survival was observed despite the fact that 72% of patients who had received chemotherapy alone crossed over at disease progression to receive Herceptin therapy. Trends indicating an increased survival benefit were also noted in patients receiving Herceptin plus paclitaxel and Herceptin plus AC relative to those receiving either paclitaxel or AC alone (table 2).

The overall survival benefit was consistent with the one-year survival incidences, which where 79 and 68% in the Herceptin plus chemotherapy group and chemotherapy alone subgroup, respectively ($p < 0.01$; table 2). Improvements in one-year survival were also noted in both Herceptin plus chemotherapy subgroups.

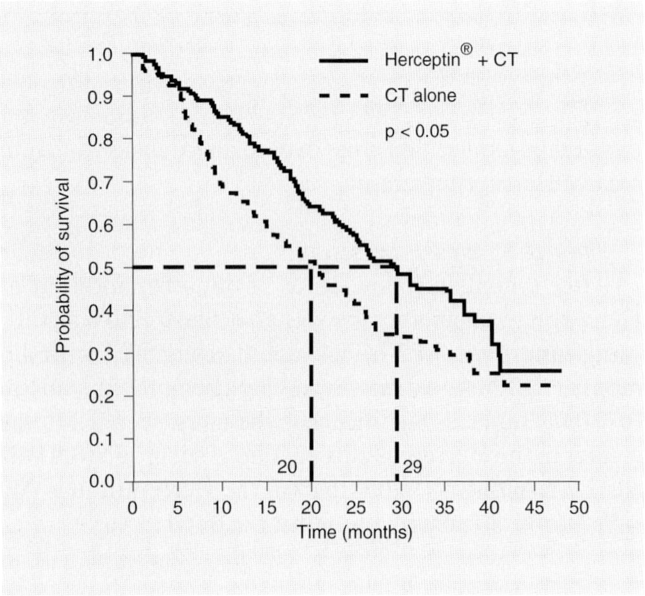

Fig. 1. Overall survival following Herceptin plus chemotherapy in IHC 3+ patients.

Subgroup Analyses

As in the pivotal phase II trial, subgroup analysis revealed that IHC 3+ patients had a greater clinical benefit from Herceptin therapy than the combined HER2 2+/3+ patient population (table 2). The median survival of HER2 3+ patients was 29 months relative to 25 months for all patients receiving Herceptin combination therapy (fig. 1). For patients receiving chemotherapy alone, the median survival was 20 months in both the overall patient population and IHC 3+ patients. Thus, adding Herceptin to chemotherapy increased survival by 45%. Increased survival benefit was also observed in IHC 3+ patients treated with either Herceptin plus paclitaxel or Herceptin plus AC, relative to IHC 2+/3+ patients receiving these treatment regimens. Small increases in the median TTP, RR, median DR and median TTF were also seen in the HER2 3+ subgroup of patients relative to all patients in the Herceptin plus paclitaxel and AC subgroups.

Outcomes for IHC 3+ and FISH-Positive Patients

IHC 3+ positivity has recently been shown to be highly concordant (89%) with FISH positivity [Mass et al. 2000]. A retrospective analysis of FISH positivity on random tissue samples from the pivotal phase III trial was performed. Analysis of patient response based on FISH status demonstrated that in FISH-negative patients response rates were similar for patients who received chemotherapy alone and Herceptin plus chemotherapy (39 and 41%, respectively). However, in FISH-positive pa-

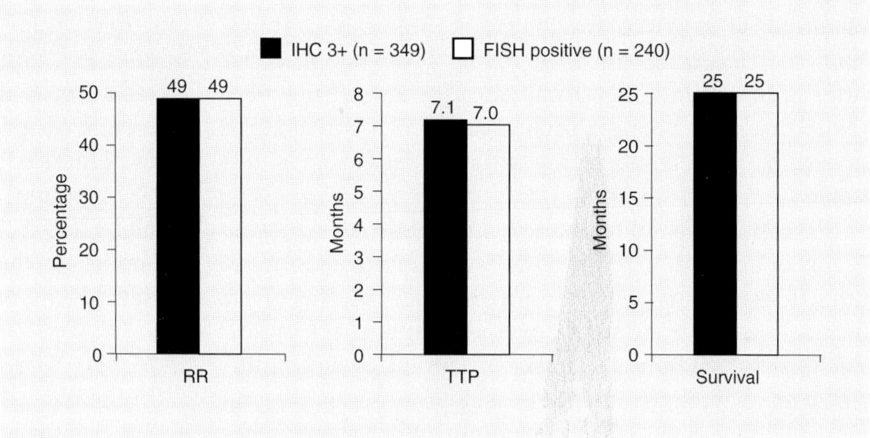

Fig. 2. Outcomes for FISH positive and IHC 3+ patients following treatment with Herceptin plus paclitaxel.

tients, response rates were significantly increased from 27% in those patients receiving chemotherapy alone to 54% in those patients receiving Herceptin plus chemotherapy.

Following retrospective analysis of FISH status in the pivotal phase III Herceptin combination trial, it was revealed that IHC 3+ and FISH-positive patients had similar clinical outcomes in terms of RR, TTP and survival following treatment with Herceptin combination therapy. For example, response rates and median survival were identical for IHC 3+ and FISH-positive patients receiving Herceptin plus paclitaxel (49% and 25 months, respectively) and median TTP was similar (7.1 versus 7.0 months for IHC 3+ and FISH-positive patients, respectively) (fig. 2). Since 24% of IHC 2+ tumors are FISH positive [Mass et al. 2000], it is probable that FISH may allow the selection of all IHC 2+ overexpressors who are likely to benefit from Herceptin therapy.

Safety

The safety profile of Herceptin in combination with chemotherapy is detailed elsewhere [Cook-Bruns 2001]. Briefly, Herceptin plus chemotherapy was generally well tolerated. Infusion-related reactions were common (approximately 40% fever and chills), but were rarely severe. These were generally associated with the first infusion and could be solved by slowing the infusion rate.

The most serious adverse event was an increased risk of cardiac dysfunction, observed in patients receiving concomitant AC. However, this was readily managed using standard medical treatment.

Conclusions

Breast cancer patients with HER2-positive tumors are known to have a poor prognosis with a reduced disease-free and overall survival [Hynes and Stern 1994; Ravdin et al. 1995; Slamon et al. 1987, 1989]. The humanized anti-HER2 MAb, Herceptin, was rationally developed to specifically target only those cells that display amplification/expression of HER2. Early clinical trials demonstrated the value of using Herceptin to treat patients with HER2-positive breast cancer who had relapsed following treatment for their metastatic disease. The pivotal phase II and phase III trials were designed to evaluate both the efficacy and safety of Herceptin when used either alone or in combination with other anticancer drugs for the treatment of HER2-positive metastatic breast cancer.

Pivotal phase II trial results demonstrate that Herceptin is active as a single agent, producing durable tumor responses. When used in combination with chemotherapy, Herceptin was associated with a significant increase in TTP, ORR, DR and TTF. These enhanced benefits with Herceptin were noted in both the paclitaxel and AC subgroups. Significantly, in the patient subgroup treated with Herceptin combined with paclitaxel, the median TTP was more than doubled (table 2).

Of particular interest is the fact that treatment of HER2-positive patients with Herceptin combined with chemotherapy in the phase III trial significantly improved overall survival compared with chemotherapy alone. This was especially evident in the IHC 3+ subsets in which patients receiving Herceptin plus either concomitant paclitaxel or AC chemotherapy demonstrated a 45% increase in overall survival after 35 months follow-up. Such a survival advantage is unusual in metastatic breast cancer. Significantly, this survival advantage was seen even though 72% of the chemotherapy alone patients crossed over to receive Herceptin after disease progression, a design that would normally bias against observing a survival advantage.

QoL has been recognized as an important issue when selecting therapy for metastatic patients. Specifically, QoL assessment enables measurement of clinical benefits and how adverse events impact on patient well being and social function [Bull et al. 1999; McLachlan et al. 1999]. Treatment with Herceptin monotherapy significantly improved the global QoL and social function of HER2-positive metastatic breast cancer patients [Lieberman et al. 1999]. Consistent with this finding is the suggestion that patients receiving Herceptin plus chemotherapy maintain their QoL, with the implication being that Herceptin may be associated with a reduction in chemotherapy-induced adverse events [Baselga et al. 1999; Osoba and Burchmore 1999].

The subset analyses of efficacy in both trials performed on the basis of IHC score revealed a clear correlation between the degree of clinical benefit obtained from Herceptin and the level of HER2 overexpression (i.e. 2+ or 3+) [Slamon et al. 2001; Roche, data on file]. Thus, although clinical responses were seen in both IHC 2+ and 3+ patients in the single agent and combination Herceptin trials, IHC 3+ patients responded better than the overall (IHC 2+/3+) patient population. Retesting of tissue samples from the pivotal trials using FISH has demonstrated that FISH positivity is highly concordant (89%) with IHC 3+ positivity. However, 24% of IHC 2+ tumors are also FISH positive. In the pivotal phase II trial no tumor responses were seen in FISH-negative patients. Moreover, in the phase III combination trial both FISH-positive and IHC 3+ patients had similar outcomes (ORR, TTP and survival) following Herceptin-containing treatment. Therefore, FISH assessment of HER2 gene amplification status may allow the most appropriate selection of patients who will benefit from Herceptin therapy, including some IHC 2+ patients.

This impact of HER2-overexpression level on clinical benefit, coupled with the similarity in outcomes between IHC 3+ and FISH-positive patients, highlights the need to accurately and reliably measure HER2 status and the importance of the HER2-testing approach used, respectively [for a review, see Hanna 2001]. Obviously, sensitive and specific HER2 testing is a prerequisite to identifying suitable candidates for Herceptin therapy and achieving maximum therapeutic benefit from Herceptin.

In conclusion, Herceptin is well tolerated and has significant efficacy in the metastatic setting, whether used as a single agent or in combination with chemotherapy. The data from the pivotal trials clearly support the important clinical benefits of Herceptin, particularly when used in combination with standard anticancer agents in the first-line treatment of patients with HER2-positive metastatic breast cancer. Moreover, the data also confirm that accurate determination of HER2 status is an essential tool for maximization of the therapeutic advantages offered by this treatment.

On the strength of the pivotal trial data demonstrating clinical efficacy and the substantially lower incidence of side effects relative to traditional cytotoxic agents, Herceptin was approved for clinical use in the USA in September 1998 [Brenner and Adams 1999]. Significantly, this represented the first approval of a humanized MAb for the treatment of breast cancer. Subsequently, Herceptin has been granted approval in a number of other countries worldwide, and the European license was granted on 28 August 2000. The clinically meaningful data generated from the pivotal trials has triggered a number of clinical trials to examine Herceptin in various regimens and combinations in the metastatic setting. Results are already emerging and appear promising [Burstein et al. 2000; Vogel et al. 2000; Winer and Burstein 2001]. Noteworthy is that the benefits of therapy appear to increase with upfront rather than delayed Herceptin usage [Cobleigh et al. 1999; Norton et al. 1999; Burstein et al. 2000; Vogel et al. 2000]. Indeed, it is predicted that Herceptin will ultimately have an important therapeutic role to play in primary breast cancer therapy [for a review, see Leyland-Jones and Smith 2001]. Trials are already at the planning stage to evaluate the applicability of Herceptin to adjuvant therapy, the results from which are awaited with interest.

References

Baselga J, Norton L, Albanell J, Kim Y-M, Mendelsohn: Recombinant humanized anti-HER2 antibody (Herceptin™) enhances the antitumor activity of paclitaxel and doxorubicin against HER2/*neu*-overexpressing human breast cancer xenografts. Cancer Res 1998;58:2825–2831.

Baselga J, Tripathy D, Mendelsohn J, Baughman S, Benz CC, Dantis L, Sklarin NT, Seidman AD, Hudis CA, Moore J, Rosen PP, Twaddell T, Henderson IC, Norton L: Phase II study of weekly intravenous recombinant humanized anti-p185^{HER2} monoclonal antibody in patients with HER/*neu*-overexpressing metastatic breast cancer. J Clin Oncol 1996;14:737–744.

Baselga J, Kerrigan M, Burchmore M, Ash M: Health-related Quality of Life (HRQL) in women with HER2-overexpressing, metastatic breast cancer (MBC) in a phase III study of Herceptin® plus chemotherapy versus chemotherapy alone. Eur J Cancer 1999;35:S318.

Brenner TL, Adams VR: First MAb approved for the treatment of metastatic breast cancer. J Am Pharm Assoc 1999;39:236–238.

Bull AA, Meyerowitz BE, Hart S, Mosconi P, Apolone G, Liberati A: Quality of life in women with recurrent breast cancer. Breast Cancer Research and Treatment 1999;54:47–57.

Burstein HJ, Kuter I, Richardson PG, Campos SM, Matulonis UA, Harris L, Garber JE, Younger J, Bunnell CA, Shulman LN, Winer EP: Herceptin (H) and Navelbine (V) for HER2-positive metastatic breast cancer: a phase II study. Proc ASCO 2000;19:102A.

Carter P, Presta L, Gorman CM, Ridgway JB, Henner D, Wong WL, Rowland AM, Kotts C, Carver ME, Shepard HM: Humanization of an anti-p185^{HER2} antibody for human cancer therapy. Proc Natl Acad Sci USA 1992;89:4285–4289.

Cobleigh MA, Vogel CL, Tripathy D, Robert NJ, Scholl S, Fehrenbacher L, Wolter JM, Paton V, Shak S, Lieberman G, Slamon DJ: Multinational study of the efficacy and safety of humanized anti-HER2 monoclonal antibody in women who have HER2-overexpressing metastatic breast cancer that has progressed after chemotherapy for metastatic disease. J Clin Oncol 1999;17:2639–2648.

Cook-Bruns N: Retrospective analysis of the safety of Herceptin® immunotherapy in metastatic breast cancer. Oncology 2001;61(suppl 2):58–66.

Coussens L, Yang-Feng TL, Liao Y-C, Chen E, Gray A, McGrath J, Seeburg PH, Libermann TA, Schlessinger J, Francke U, et al: Tyrosine kinase receptor with extensive homology to EGF receptor shares chromosomal location with neu oncogene. Science 1985;230:1132–1139.

Di Fiore PP, Pierce JH, Fleming TP, Hazan R, Ullrich A, King CR, Schlessinger J, Aaronson SA: Overexpression of the human EGF receptor confers an EGF-dependent transformed phenotype to NIH 3T3 cells. Cell 1987a;51:1063–1070.

Di Fiore PP, Pierce JH, Kraus MH, Segatto O, King CR, Aaronson SA: *erb*B-2 is a potent oncogene when overexpressed in NIH/3T3 cells. Science 1987b;237:178–182.

Guy CT, Webster MA, Schaller M, Parsons TJ, Cardiff RD, Muller WJ: Expression of the *neu* protooncogene in the mammary epithelium of transgenic mice includes metastatic disease. Proc Natl Acad Sci USA 1992;89:10578–10582.

Hancock MC, Langton BC, Chan T, Toy P, Monahan JJ, Mischak RP, Shawver LK: A monoclonal antibody against the C-erbB-2 protein enhances the cytotoxicity of cis-diamminedichloroplatinum against human breast and ovarian tumor cell lines. Cancer Res 1991;51: 4575–4580.

Hanna W: Testing for HER2 status. Oncology 2001;61(suppl 2):22–30.

Hudziak RM, Lewis GD, Winget M, Fendley BM, Shepard HM, Ullrich A: p185HER2 monoclonal antibody has antiproliferative effects in vitro and sensitizes human breast tumor cells to tumor necrosis factor. Mol Cell Biol 1989;9: 1165–1172.

Hudziak RM, Schlessinger J, Ullrich A: Increased expression of the putative growth factor receptor $p185^{HER2}$ causes transformation and tumorigenesis of NIH 3T3 cells. Proc Natl Acad Sci USA 1987;84:7159–7163.

Hynes NE, Stern DF: The biology of *erb*B-2/*neu*/*HER*-2 and its role in cancer. Biochim Biophys Acta Rev Cancer 1994;1198:165–184.

Lewis GD, Figari I, Fendley B, Wong WL, Carter P, Gorman C, Shepard HM: Differential responses of human tumor cell lines to anti-p185HER2 monoclonal antibodies. Cancer Immunol Immunother 1993;37:255–263.

Leyland-Jones B, Smith I: Role of Herceptin® in primary breast cancer: Views from North America and Europe. Oncology 2001;61(suppl 2):83–91.

Lieberman G, Burchmore MJ, Ferhenbacher L, Cobleigh M: Health related quality of life (HRQL) of patients with HER-2 overexpressing, metastatic breast cancer (MBC) treated with Herceptin (Trastuzumab) as a single agent. Proc Am Soc Clin Oncol 1999;18:417A.

Mass RD, Sanders C, Charlene K, Everett T, Johnson L, Anderson S: The concordance between the clinical trials assay (CTA) and fluorescence in situ hybridization (FISH) in the Herceptin pivotal trials. Proc Am Soc Clin Oncol 2000; 19:75A.

McKenzie SJ, Marks PJ, Lam T, Morgan J, Panicali DL, Trimpe KL, Carney WP: Generation and characterization of monoclonal antibodies specific for the human neu oncogene product, p185. Oncogene 1989;4:543–548.

McLachlan SA, Pintilie M, Tannock IF: Third line chemotherapy in patients with metastatic breast cancer: an evaluation of quality of life and cost. Breast Cancer Res Treat 1999;54: 313–323.

Ménard S, Fortis S, Castiglioni F, Agresti R, Balsari A: HER2 as a prognostic factor in breast cancer. Oncology 2001;61(suppl 2):67–72.

Norton L, Slamon D, Leyland-Jones B Wolter J, Fleming T, Eirmann W, Baselga J, Mendelsohn J, Bajamonde A, Ash M, Shak S: Overall survival (OS) advantage to simultaneous chemotherapy (CRx) plus the humanized anti-HER2 monoclonal antibody Herceptin (H) in HER2-overexpressing (HER2+) metastatic breast cancer (MBC). Proc Am Soc Clin Oncol 1999;18: 127A.

Osoba D, Burchmore M: Health-related quality of life in women with metastatic breast cancer treated with trastuzumab (Herceptin). Semin Oncol 1999;26(suppl 12):84–88.

Pegram MD, Lipton A, Hayes DF, Weber BL, Baselga JM, Tripathy D, Baly D, Baughman SA, Twaddell T, Glaspy JA, Slamon DJ: Phase II study of receptor-enhanced chemosensitivity using recombinant humanized anti-$p185^{HER2/neu}$ monoclonal antibody plus cisplatin in patients with HER2/*neu*-overexpressing metastatic breast cancer refractory to chemotherapy treatment. J Clin Oncol 1998;16:2659–2671.

Ravdin PM, Chamness GC. The *c-erbB*-2 protooncogene as a prognostic and predictive marker in breast cancer: a paradigm for the development of other macromolecular markers – a review. Gene 1995;159:19–27.

Slamon D, Leyland-Jones B, Shak S, Paton V, Bajamonde A, Fleming T, Eirmann W, Wolter J, Baselga J, Norton L: Addition of Herceptin™ (humanized anti-HER2 antibody) to first line chemotherapy for HER2 overexpressing metastatic breast cancer (HER2+/MBC) markedly increases anticancer activity: a randomized multinational controlled phase III trial. Proc Am Soc Clin Oncol 1998;17:98A.

Slamon DJ, Clark GM, Wong SG Levin WJ, Ullrich A, McGuire WL: Human breast cancer: correlation of relapse and survival with amplification of the HER-2/*neu* oncogene. Science 1987;235:177–182.

Slamon DJ, Godolphin W, Jones LA, Holt JA, Wong SG, Keith DE, Levin WJ, Stuart SG, Udove J, Ullrich A, Press MF: Studies of the HER2/*neu* proto-oncogene in human breast and ovarian cancer. Science 1989;244:707–712.

Slamon DJ, Leyland-Jones B, Shak S, Fuchs H, Paton V, Bajamonde A, Fleming T, Eiermann W, Wolter J, Pegram M, Baselga J, Norton L: Use of chemotherapy plus a monoclonal antibody against HER2 for metastatic breast cancer that overexpresses HER2. N Engl J Med 2001;344:783–792.

Stancovski I, Hurwltz E, Leitner O, Ullrich A, Yarden Y, Sela M: Mechanistic aspects of the opposing effects of monoclonal antibodies to the erbB2 receptor on tumor growth. Proc Natl Acad Sci USA 1991;88:8691–8695.

Vogel C, Cobleigh M, Tripathy D, Harris L, Fehrenbacher L, Slamon D, Ash M, Novotny W, Stewart S, Shak S: First-line, non-hormonal, treatment of woman with HER2 overexpressing metastatic breast cancer with Herceptin (trastuzumab, humanized anti-HER2 antibody). Proc Am Soc Clin Oncol 2000;19:71A.

Winer EP, Burstein HJ: New combinations with Herceptin® in metastatic breast cancer. Oncology 2001;61(suppl 2):50–57.

Oncology

Oncology 2001;61(suppl 2):22–30

Testing for HER2 Status

Wedad Hanna

Sunnybrook and Women's College Health Sciences Centre, Toronto, Ont., Canada

Key Words

HER2 testing · Fluorescence in situ hybridization · Immunohistochemistry · Polymerase chain reaction · Validate · Correspondence · Standardization

Abstract

Incorporation of a new biological marker such as HER2 into routine clinical practice requires proof that it provides reproducible information independent of, and better than, conventional pathologic criteria, and that it influences treatment decisions. In breast cancer, HER2 amplification/overexpression predicts for a poor clinical outcome and an enhanced survival benefit from the HER2-targeted therapy, Herceptin®, and may predict for resistance to some conventional therapies. Thus, HER2 is considered to be a clinically important molecule and testing for HER2 abnormalities is already part of routine patient assessment in many parts of the world. There is currently no gold standard for HER2 testing. The main challenge is to standardize and technically validate HER2 testing methodologies. Immunohistochemistry (IHC) and fluorescence in situ hybridization (FISH) are the most common HER2 tests used, and show a high level of concordance. HER2 testing approaches based on the polymerase chain reaction (PCR) are under extensive investigation and appear promising. A Canadian HER2 testing algorithm designed to increase the validity and reproducibility of HER2 testing has been compiled. HER2-positive cases are defined as those with >10% of tumor cells with moderate/strong, complete membrane staining in the invasive component, by IHC. Confirmatory HER2 testing using either FISH or quantitative PCR is recommended for indeterminate cases. Additional studies are required to calibrate HER2 testing results to clinical outcome.

Introduction

Pathologists play a pivotal role in the evaluation of prognostic and predictive factors that guide treatment and management decisions in breast cancer. In addition to morphologic factors such as axillary lymph node status, tumor size, histologic grade and lymphovascular invasion, molecular markers measured in the tumor or serum provide prognostic and/or predictive information that enables optimization of treatment selection for, and management of, breast cancer patients [for a review, see Hanna et al., 1999; Piccart et al., 2001; Ménard et al., 2001; Ross and Fletcher 1998]. Thus, markers help clinicians to determine the recurrence probability and expected treatment benefit/risk ratio. Markers with a predictive index are especially clinically relevant in that they enable tailored treatment selection.

Several groups of clinicians, pathologists and statisticians have used various categorical ranking and tumor-marker grading systems to stratify prognostic and predictive factors in breast cancer according to the strength of published evidence regarding their clinical utility [ASCO 1998; Fitzgibbons et al. 2000; Henson et al. 1994; Hayes

KARGER

Fax +41 61 306 12 34
E-Mail karger@karger.ch
www.karger.com

0030–2414/01/0616–0022$17.50/0

Accessible online at:
www.karger.com/journals/ocl

Wedad Hanna, MB, BCh, FRCP
Department of Pathology, Sunnybrook and Women's College Health Sciences Centre
University of Toronto, 76 Grenville Street
Toronto, Ont. M5S 1B2 (Canada)
Tel. +1 416 323 6142, Fax +1 416 323 6116, E-Mail wedad.hanna@swchsc.on.ca

et al. 1996, 1998; McGuire 1991; Piccart et al. 1999]. For example, the College of American Pathologists recognizes three categories of marker [Fitzgibbons et al. 2000]. Category I comprises factors proven to be of prognostic importance and useful in clinical patient management, category II contains factors that have been extensively studied biologically and clinically, but whose importance remains to be validated in statistically robust studies, and category III is made up of all other factors not sufficiently studied to demonstrate their prognostic utility. Although there are minor differences among the various sets of published guidelines, they all agree that, in order to be useful, a marker must be validated both clinically and technically and also be capable of influencing treatment decisions. At the clinical level, the marker must identify subsets of patients with significantly different risks of relapse, survival or response to therapy. Ideally, the predictive power of the marker should be proven to be reproducible in multiple large studies of randomized patients.

Although the issue of validating tumor markers has received considerable attention in recent years, very few have actually been validated clinically and technically for routine clinical assessment in breast cancer. At present, the only validated factors are estrogen receptor (ER) and progesterone receptor, both of which predict for a response to hormonal therapy.

HER2 as a Prognostic/Predictive Marker

The human epidermal growth factor receptor-2 (HER2) is amplified/overexpressed in 20–30% of breast cancer patients [Slamon et al. 1987, 1989]. HER2 overexpression is the result of gene amplification and/or enhanced transcription, whereas gene amplification results from an increased number of gene copies per chromosome or aneuploidy [Hynes and Stern 1994; Pauletti et al. 1996; Vona et al. 1999]. Current evidence supports a clear association between HER2 amplification/overexpression and a reduced overall and disease-free survival, especially in patients with node-positive disease [Hynes 1993; Hynes and Stern 1994; Slamon et al. 1987, 1989].

Studies have also emerged to indicate a predictive role for HER2 in response to some therapeutic regimens [for a review, see Dowsett et al. 2000; Piccart et al., 2001; Ross and Fletcher 1998]. Most noteworthy are the results from large, randomized clinical trials [Cobleigh et al. 1999; Norton et al. 1999; Slamon et al. 1998, 2001], which have shown that metastatic breast cancer patients with HER2-positive tumors obtain an enhanced survival benefit from the humanized monoclonal anti-HER2 antibody, Herceptin®. Furthermore, HER2 positivity also appears to predict for resistance to treatment with cyclophosphamide, methotrexate and 5-FU (CMF), endocrine therapy and tamoxifen [for a review, see Piccart et al., 2001].

Despite the substantial evidence to support the prognostic and predictive power of HER2 with respect to certain therapies, controversy still surrounds the clinical usefulness of HER2 [Dowsett et al. 2000]. This is reflected by the assignment of a category II ranking to HER2 by the College of American Pathologists [Fitzgibbons et al. 2000]. The American Society of Clinical Oncology (ASCO) guidelines on the use of tumor markers cite the potential predictive value of HER2 as its most clinically relevant use [ASCO 1998]. Their 2000 update on the predictive index of HER2 notes that high levels of HER2 expression or HER2 amplification can be used to identify patients for whom Herceptin may be of benefit for the treatment of metastatic, recurrent, and/or treatment-refractory unresectable locally advanced breast cancer [Bast et al. 2001]. There is also a growing consensus that HER2 is approaching a clinically validated status as a prognostic factor as well as a predictive factor for response to some systemic therapies. This acknowledgement of the clinical relevance of HER2 means that HER2 testing should be part of the routine assessment for breast cancer patients. Indeed, of the other markers recently considered by ASCO for use in breast cancer, including p53, cathepsin-D, carcinoembryonic antigen and CA-15-3, determination of HER2 status is the only one recommended for routine use [Bast et al. 2001]. The authors state that HER2 status should be evaluated on every primary breast cancer at the time of diagnosis or at the time of recurrence.

Validation of HER2 Testing

The recent increase in the use of HER2 testing of current and archived breast tumor specimens to obtain prognostic and predictive information has greatly heightened the pressure to obtain technical validation of HER2 testing. Technical validation means that the testing assay is sensitive, specific, reproducible, can be interpreted in a relatively uniform manner between laboratories and, importantly, that the technical validation has been calibrated to clinical outcome. Lack of standardization and inaccuracy in HER2 test results may lead to inappropriate patient evaluation and therapy selection [Hanna et al. 1999; Nelson 2000]. Obviously, specific and reliable determination of HER2 status has direct implications for the appropriate use of Herceptin. As discussed below, numerous programs are ongoing at national and international levels to compare and validate HER2 testing methodologies.

The majority of published reports examining the impact of HER2 status on clinical outcome and response to therapy employed retrospective HER2 testing, primarily by immunohistochemistry (IHC). This feature has, in part, contributed to the difficulty experienced in obtaining a consensus regarding the prognostic/predictive index of HER2. However, it is now clear that HER2 status should be measured prospectively in order to apply its prognostic and predictive value to guide therapy selection. Routine testing for HER2 status at presentation avoids having to retrieve histologic blocks. Furthermore, archival tissues can be accessed in the metastatic setting, if required.

HER2 Testing Methods

A major issue among pathologists and oncologists is the current lack of agreement as to the best approach to measure HER2 status [for a review, see Dowsett et al. 2000; Allred et al. 2000]. Unfortunately, a wide variety of non-standardized methods that target either HER2 overexpression or HER2 amplification are available worldwide. Moreover, a large number of pathology laboratories use in-house reagents and protocols with widely varying sensitivity, specificity, reproducibility and practicability.

HER2 testing methodologies measure HER2 overexpression at the DNA level by fluorescence in situ hybridization (FISH), Southern blot [Tandon et al. 1989; Thor et al. 1989] and polymerase chain reaction (PCR), which can be competitive [Deng et al. 1999; Okuyama et al. 1999; Vona et al. 1999], differential [Deng et al. 1999; Frye et al. 1989; Gramlich et al. 1994] or real-time PCR [Bieche et al. 1999; Higuchi et al. 1993]; at the RNA level by Northern blot [Slamon et al. 1989]; or at the protein level by IHC, enzyme-linked immunosorbent assay (ELISA) and Western blot [Slamon et al. 1989]. Some of these methods require resources and expertise exceeding those available in the average pathology laboratory and preclude the use of archival material. Therefore, FISH and IHC performed on sections cut from formalin-fixed, paraffin-embedded specimens have emerged as the most frequently employed techniques in clinical practice and clinical research studies.

IHC

IHC employs an antibody to probe for HER2 in tumor cells. The HER2 protein is visualized by attaching a color-emitting molecule. Approximately 75% of pathologists currently use IHC, making it the dominant HER2 testing method [Allred et al. 2000]. Surprisingly, more than 30 anti-HER2 mouse monoclonal or rabbit/goat polyclonal antibodies are available. These antibodies display widely differing sensitivities and specificities and are directed towards either the extracellular or intramembraneous domains of the HER2 receptor. A definite advantage of IHC over other testing technologies is that it can be performed easily on formalin-fixed, paraffin-embedded tissue, which is the form in which tissue from clinical trials is typically preserved, as well as on frozen samples.

Given the suitability of IHC to formalin-fixed, paraffin-embedded tissue, the reports published on the clinical relevance of HER2 were performed almost exclusively using IHC on paraffin blocks [for a review, see Ross and Fletcher 1998]. In a retrospective study [Press et al. 1994] of 187 archival paraffin-embedded breast cancer tissues with known HER2 amplification/overexpression status, the sensitivity of 28 different anti-HER2 antibodies was assessed. Depending on the antibody used, a sensitivity of 6–82% was obtained. Importantly, only immunostaining of cell membranes was found to correlate with HER2 overexpression; staining of tumor cell cytoplasm or nuclei and staining of noncarcinoma cells was not associated with HER2 positivity. These observations led the authors to conclude that the variability in sensitivity in archival tissues is likely to have been a major factor contributing to the widely differing HER2 immunostaining incidences reported in the literature.

Differences in antibody sensitivity are, however, not solely responsible for the reported disparity in HER2 testing results. Tissue fixation and processing, as well as differences in scoring criteria, controls and interobserver variability in interpreting results can all contribute to variability. The potential of the fixative used to influence staining has been documented [Penault-Llorca et al. 1994]. Although alcoholic formalin is superior to phosphate-buffered formalin and preserves the tissue better, it is more expensive and not commonly used. In addition, the widespread use of Bouin's stain in Europe is not ideal because it may make retrospective testing difficult. Antigen masking may also occur, depending on the duration and type of fixative used. Antigen retrieval, which is practiced in some but not all laboratories and is achieved by protease digestion or heat treatment in citrate buffer, may

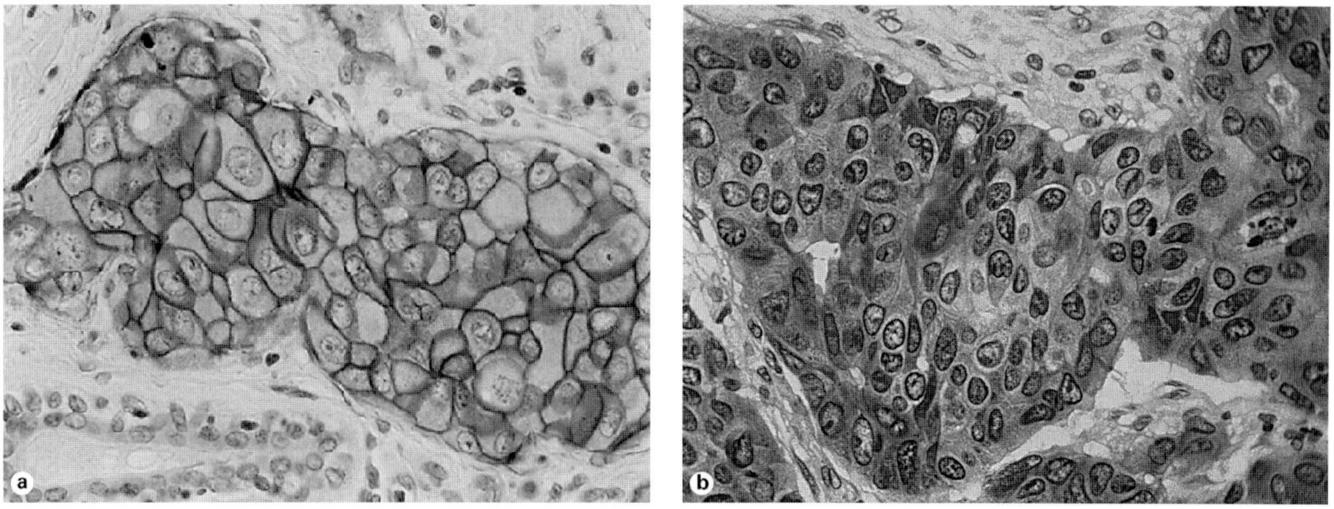

Fig. 1. Issues when interpreting IHC-stained sections for HER2. **a** Complete membrane staining. **b** Cytoplasmic staining.

increase the incidence of HER2 positivity unrelated to the level of HER2 amplification [Farabegoli et al. 1999]. Another confounding issue is the duration of storage of unstained slides. It has been reported that prolonged storage of unstained slides can result in significant loss of immunostaining intensity for some antigens/antibodies [Jacobs et al. 1996]. To date, there have been no reports of this relating to HER2.

When interpreting and scoring IHC-stained slides, the percentage of positively staining cells, the intensity and location (cytoplasmic versus membranous and ductal carcinoma in situ versus invasive component) of staining, and the positivity cut-off used are all important factors (fig. 1). In particular, different positivity cut-offs are in use. For example, a Cancer and Leukemia Group B (CALGB) study employed a dichotomous HER2 scoring system in which <50% and >50% of cells with membrane staining were scored as low and high HER2 expression, respectively [Thor et al. 1998]. In contrast, a recent National Adjuvant Surgical Breast and Bowel Project (NSABP) study interpreted HER2 positivity as being any membrane staining [Paik et al. 1998]. The subjective nature of interpreting the intensity of IHC staining represents a particular inherent weakness with IHC. The issue of interobserver variability of HER2 IHC interpretation has been examined by Kay and coworkers [1994]. They found that there was a high (89%) level of agreement with regard to the presence or absence of membrane staining, but a low (40%) level of agreement with intensity and extent of tumor membrane staining. However, one recent report has indicated excellent interlaboratory agreement for HER2 testing using the same primary antibody to HER2, even without standardization of the assay method or scoring criteria [Jacobs et al. 2000]. Clearly, the use of standardized references and scoring systems have an important role to play in the minimization of interobserver variation. At present, laboratories employ stained cell lines or tissue sections as references for HER2 testing. An automated cellular imaging instrument such as ChromaVision enables the pathologist to quickly obtain quantitative reproducible results from stained sections and eliminates the inherent subjectivity associated with current IHC procedures [Hatanaka et al. 2001]. At present, however, this type of instrument remains prohibitively expensive.

Given the considerable variability among the results obtained with the variety of IHC testing protocols currently used, a standardized IHC-based HER2 test offers clear benefits. Only one commercially available IHC-based HER2-testing kit, HercepTest (DAKO), has received US Food and Drug Administration (FDA) approval for clinical use. This kit offers several advantages, including a comprehensive protocol, standardized reagents and control slides. A numeric score ranging from 0 to 3 that reflects the staining intensity and pattern in 10% or more of tumor cells is employed. Although relatively expensive, the HercepTest is popular because of its convenience and standardized format. However, several reports have emerged in criticism of the arbitrary and oversimplified nature of its scoring system, which has been reported to overestimate HER2 positivity levels [Jacobs et al. 1999b; Maia 1999; Roche and Ingle 1999]. Using the HercepTest to assess 48 breast cancers previously shown to be HER2 negative by two different IHC assays and FISH, Jacobs and colleagues [Jacobs et al. 1999b] reported that the HercepTest had a low specificity and produced many apparently false positives. A modified scoring system that takes into account the level of staining of non-neoplastic epithelium was found to provide greater specificity. However, at least one report has indicated that the HercepTest produces HER2 positivity rates within the expected range of 20–30% and with good concordance between FISH and an in-house IHC test [Espinoza et al. 1999]. Additional studies to define the sensitivity of the HercepTest are clearly warranted.

FISH

FISH, which measures gene amplification, is the second most common HER2 testing technique and is a highly sensitive (96.5%) approach [Pauletti et al. 1996], with a remarkable 100% specificity. In addition to its sensitivity and reproducibility, FISH, unlike IHC, offers an entirely objective and quantitative measurement of HER2 abnormalities. However, distinct disadvantages are the loss of physical linkage between the centromere and chromosome of interest, signal heterogeneity due to nuclear truncation, intrachromosomal amplification versus double minute chromosome as well as its cost, the need for specialist equipment, and time and skills for interpretation. For these reasons, the use of FISH is currently relatively limited, although its advantages and its capacity for automation are certain to boost future usage.

Two FDA-approved FISH kits are currently available. The Inform HER2 Kit (ONCOR/Ventana) uses a single probe to measure the absolute number of HER2 gene copies. In contrast, the more popular PathVysion™ Kit (Vysis™) uses two DNA probes; one specifically recognizes the HER2 gene and the other is specific for the chromosome 17 centromere. Gene and centromere signals are determined in 60 nuclei and the HER2 gene:chromosome 17 centromere ratio is calculated. A ratio of ≥ 2 indicates HER2 amplification. This kit has recently been reported to yield a high level of interlaboratory reproducibility for HER2 testing of formalin-fixed, paraffin-embedded breast cancer samples with different levels of amplification [Persons et al. 2000].

FISH/IHC Concordance

Given that some laboratories prefer IHC while others opt for FISH, it was important to establish the degree of concordance between testing results obtained with these two techniques. A high level of concordance (typically 90%) is obtained between FISH and IHC [Jacobs et al. 1999a, 2000; Jiminez et al. 2000], with <5% of breast tumors showing HER2 overexpression in the absence of HER2 amplification. Consistent with this observation, FISH has been shown to have a high (82%) level of concordance with the clinical trials assay (CTA) [Mass et al. 2000] , the test used to identify HER2-positive patients for the Herceptin pivotal trials. This assay employed the MAbs CB11 and 4D5 and patients with an IHC score of 2+ or 3+ by either antibody were enrolled into the trial. In cases where both antibodies were used, the higher score was taken. In patients whose tumors displayed substantial HER2 overexpression (IHC 3+), the level of concordance with FISH was 89%.

FDA approval was granted to the HercepTest on the strength of its 79% concordance with the CTA. It is noteworthy, however, that this concordance analysis was performed using more than 500 breast tumors unrelated to those tested for the Herceptin clinical trials. Significantly, 42% of IHC 2+ results obtained using the HercepTest tested negative (0 to 1+) using the CTA, indicating that the HercepTest may be too sensitive, as discussed above. Thus, had these patients been tested with the CTA, they would not have been considered candidates for Herceptin therapy. Unlike the CTA, there have been no reports to date correlating HercepTest results with clinical outcome. Studies comparing the HercepTest with other more established IHC assays are imminent and should further define its clinical usefulness.

Both FISH and IHC provide biologically and clinically useful information and research has suggested that a combination of the two methods may be beneficial [Ratcliffe et al. 1997]. However, the potential usefulness and practicality of this dual method has yet to be defined.

PCR

Recent years have seen an increase in the number of studies devoted to evaluating the role of PCR to quantitatively measure HER2 amplification in breast cancer [Gramlich et al. 1994; Youngson et al. 1995]. Differential PCR targets the HER2 gene and a reference gene, enabling calculation of a ratio of PCR products of the target gene to the reference gene (fig. 2). This approach is easy to perform on paraffin blocks and is readily interpreted either visually or by semi-quantitative or quantitative densitometry [Frye et al. 1989; Gramlich et al. 1994]. However, its drawbacks are that it is time-consuming, tedious and expensive. Competitive PCR is another suitable HER2 testing option that has received increasing attention recently [Deng et al. 1999; Okuyama et al. 1999; Vona et al. 1999].

An alternative technology particularly suited to a reference laboratory that performs quality assurance is real-time PCR, which quantitates DNA or RNA by monitoring the products of PCR during the PCR process [Higuchi et al. 1993]. This is a powerful tool for HER2 testing for large randomized, prospective cooperative group trials [Bieche et al. 1999]. Although costly, real-time PCR is performed in a high-throughput format within a closed-tube system, thereby offering greater convenience and minimal sample contamination.

Quantitative detection of HER2 in tumors is often hampered by the mixture of non-neoplastic bystander and stroma cells. Laser microdissection has been used in conjunction with real-time PCR to overcome this obstacle and to develop an objective quantitative method. This combined approach is suitable for archival tissue specimens and should enable the exact quantification of gene copy numbers, even in small and precancerous tumors [Lehmann et al. 2000].

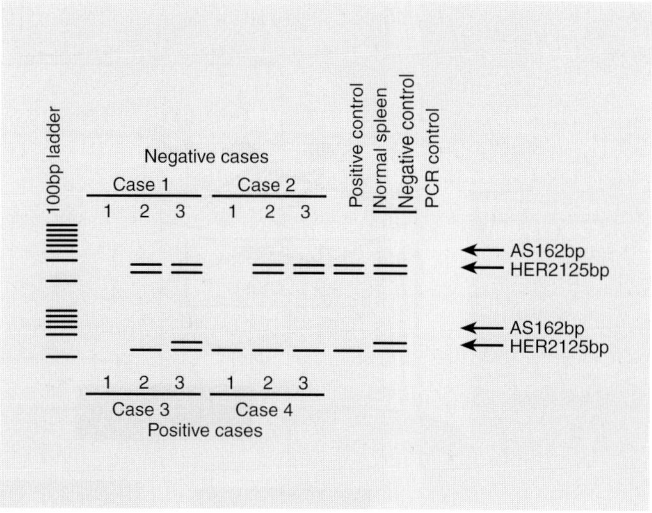

Fig. 2. HER2 amplification by differential PCR.

Clinical Validation of HER2 Testing

Calibrating HER2 testing results to clinical outcome is an immediate need. Clinical outcome data are already available for the CTA. The pivotal phase II and phase III trials to evaluate single-agent Herceptin and Herceptin in combination with chemotherapy, respectively, revealed a significantly greater clinical benefit from Herceptin plus chemotherapy in patients with an IHC score of 3+ versus those with IHC 2+ HER2 overexpression [Cobleigh et al. 1999; Mass et al. 2000]. This higher level of efficacy in patients with considerable HER2 overexpression has been confirmed in a trial of single-agent Herceptin as first-line therapy [Vogel et al. 2000, 2001].

Canadian HER2 Testing Algorithm

The availability of Herceptin via a Special Access Program in Canada since January 1999, the absence of funding for the HercepTest in that country (until January, 2001), coupled with the global need to standardize and validate HER2 testing has prompted the establishment of a Canadian HER2 testing algorithm (fig. 3). A series of collaborative workshops attended by pathologists from all 10 Canadian provinces provided a forum at which to critically examine the clinically and technically validated data available for HER2. These meetings culminated in a series of specific recommendations drawn up to assist pathologists in testing for HER2. Of the spectrum of anti-HER2 MAbs available, the use of the more commonly used and better characterized anti-HER2 MAbs CB11 (Novocastra), Tab250 (Zymed Laboratories) or A0485 (DAKO; alone or in the HercepTest) was recommended. A positive tissue control and, if possible, cell lines demonstrating high, intermediate and low-level HER2 amplification/overexpression and an internal negative control were also recommended. The guidelines drawn up by the Canadian pathologists define HER2-positive cases as those with >10% tumor cells with moderate/strong, complete membrane staining in the invasive component, as tested using IHC with the recommended antibodies. In indeterminate cases, confirmatory HER2 testing using either FISH or quantitative PCR is recommended. If differential PCR is performed, a case is interpreted as HER2 positive if ≥ 2 gene copies are detected. The Vysis™ probe is recommended for FISH, with FISH positivity constituting a ratio of the HER2 signal to chromosome 17 signal of ≥ 2.

Due to the high variability in HER2 testing approaches in current usage, it is particularly important that all

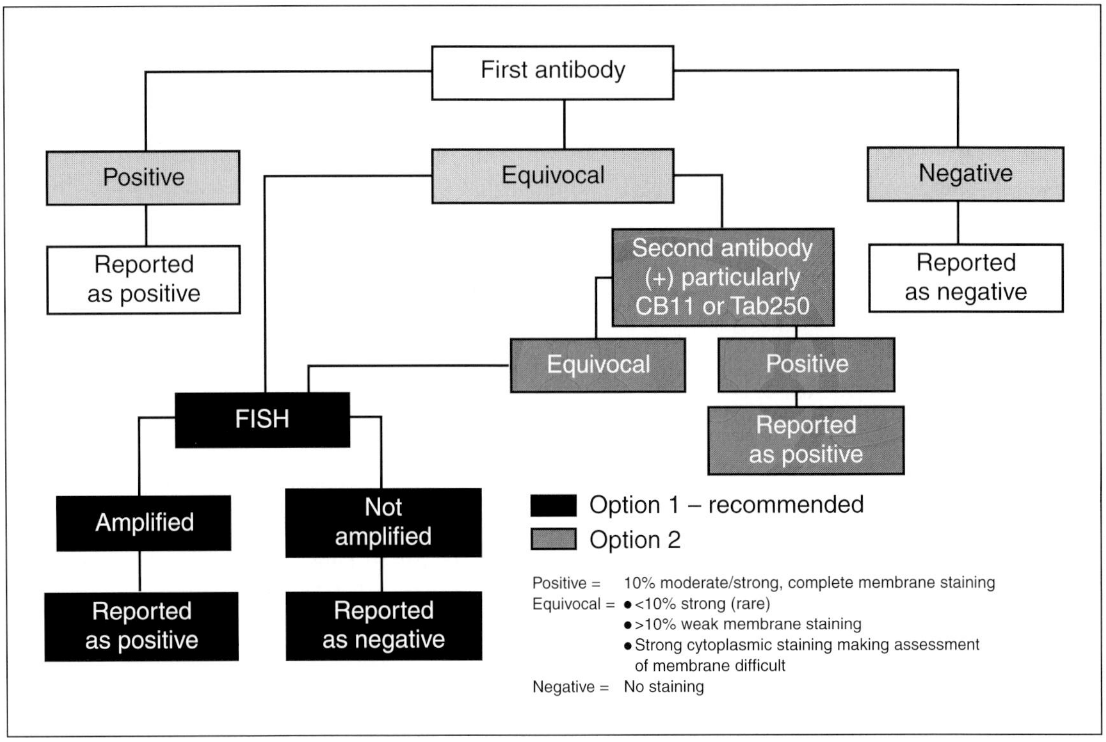

Fig. 3. Canadian HER2 testing algorithm. These guidelines are under continual review by the Canadian Pathologists' Working Party. Roche Canada facilitated the process of bringing the Canadian pathologists together to generate this algorithm.

details of the HER2 testing protocol and reagents used should be cited in full when reporting HER2 testing results. Only with accurate and complete records of testing methods can useful and valid comparisons between studies be made. A number of HER2 testing quality control initiatives are underway worldwide to increase the reproducibility of HER2 testing. As in other countries, Canada is conducting an interlaboratory program to validate HER2 testing procedures. This project involves HER2 testing of 30 tissue samples in 20 laboratories across Canada [O'Malley et al. 2001].

Conclusions

Knowledge of HER2 status provides prognostic and predictive information in breast cancer, with the result that HER2 testing has become part of the routine assessment for breast cancer patients. Correct identification of patients with HER2-positive tumors is necessary not only to identify those patients likely to have a shortened disease-free and overall survival but also to select appropriate candidates for Herceptin therapy. The increased demand for HER2 testing to enable better treatment selection and patient management has been further heightened by the recent availability of Herceptin. However, a major concern with current HER2 testing is the widespread use of different methods and a general lack of standardization between methods. The most common HER2 testing approaches are IHC and FISH, which have been reported to have a high degree of fidelity. Although IHC is readily available in most pathology laboratories, HER2 testing results are widely variable and influenced by several factors, including the antibody, fixative and scoring system used. One US FDA-approved IHC kit, the HercepTest, is commercially available, the sensitivity of which requires further clarification. In contrast to IHC, FISH is highly sensitive and reproducible, but has the drawback of being expensive and requiring specialist expertise and expensive equipment. Automation of the existing as well as emerging PCR-based HER2 testing approaches is expected to play an increasing role in future HER2 testing.

In view of the current lack of a gold standard for HER2 testing, the importance of obtaining accurate and reliable results with current HER2 testing methods, and the availability of Herceptin for HER2-positive breast cancer patients, Canadian pathologists have devised a HER2 testing algorithm. This identifies HER2-positive cases as those with >10% of tumor cells with moderate/strong, complete membrane staining in the invasive component. Confirmatory HER2 testing using either FISH or quantitative PCR is recommended for indeterminate cases. In response to the need for greater clinical and technical validation of HER2 testing, numerous quality control initiatives are underway worldwide to increase accuracy and reproducibility in HER2 testing. To facilitate comparability between studies, it is essential that all details of the HER2 testing protocol and reagents used should be cited in full when reporting HER2 testing results.

References

Allred DC, Swanson PE: Testing for erbB-2 by immunohistochemistry in breast cancer. Am J Clin Pathol 2000;113:171–175.

American Society of Clinical Oncology (ASCO): 1997 uptake of the recommendations of the use of tumour markers in breast and colorectal cancer. J Clin Oncol 1998;16:793–795.

Bast RC Jr, Ravdin P, Hayes DF, Bates S, Fritsche H Jr, Jessup JM, Kemeny N, Locker GY, Mennel RG, Somerfield MR: 2000 update of recommendations for the use of tumor markers in breast and colorectal cancer: clinical practice guidelines of the American Society of Clinical Oncology. J Clin Oncol 2001;19:1865–1878.

Bieche I, Onody P, Laurendeau I, Olivi M, Vidaud D, Lidereau R, Vidaud M: Real-time reverse transcription-PCR assay for future management of ERBB2-based clinical applications. Clin Chem 1999;45:1148–1156.

Cobleigh MA, Vogel CL, Tripathy D, Robert NJ, Scholl S, Fehrenbacher L, Wolter JM, Paton V, Shak S, Lieberman G, Slamon DJ: Multinational study of the efficacy and safety of humanized anti-HER2 monoclonal antibody in women who have HER2-overexpressing metastatic breast cancer that has progressed after chemotherapy for metastatic disease. J Clin Oncol 1999;17:2639–2648.

Deng G, Kim YS: Quantitation of erb-B-2 gene copy number in breast cancer by an improved polymerase chain reaction (PCR) technique, competitively differential PCR. Breast Cancer Res Treat 1999;58:213–217.

Dowsett M, Cooke T, Ellis I, Gullick WJ, Gusterson B, Ballon E, Mallon E, Walker R: Assessment of HER2 status in breast cancer: why, when and how? Eur J Cancer 2000:36:160–176.

Espinoza F, Anguiano A: The HercepTest assay: another perspective. J Clin Oncol 1999;17: 2293–2294.

Farabegoli F, Ceccarelli C, Santini D, Baldini N, Tafurelli M, Marrano D, Trere D, Derenzini M: c-erbB-2 overexpression in amplified and non-amplified breast carcinoma samples. Int J Cancer 1999;84:273–277.

Fitzgibbons PL, Page DL, Weaver D, Thor AD, Allred DC, Clark GM, Ruby SG, O'Malley F, Simpson JF, Connolly JL, Hayes DF, Edge SB, Lichter A, Schnitt SJ: Prognostic Factors in Breast Cancer. Arch Pathol Lab Med 2000;124: 966–978.

Frye RA, Benz CC, Liu E: Detection of amplified oncogenes by differential polymerase chain reaction. Oncogene 1989;4:1153–1157.

Gramlich TL, Cohen C, Fritsch C, DeRose PB, Gansler T: Evaluation of c-erbB-2 amplification in breast carcinoma by differential polymerase chain reaction. Am J Clin Pathol 1994; 101:493–494.

Hanna W, Kahn HJ, Trudeau M: Evaluation of HER-2/neu (erbB-2) status in breast cancer: from bench to bedside. Mol Pathol 1999;12: 827–834.

Hatanaka Y, Hashizume K, Kamihara Y, Itoh H, Tsuda H, Yoshiyuki Osamura R, Tani Y: Quantitative immunohistochemical evaluation of HER2/neu expression with HercepTest in breast carcinoma by image analysis. Pathol Internat 2001;51:33–36.

Hayes DF, Bast R, Desch CE: A tumor marker utility grading system (TMUGS): a framework to evaluate clinical utility of tumor markers. J Natl Cancer Inst 1996;88:1456–1466.

Hayes DF, Trock B, Harris AL: Assessing the clinical impact of prognostic factors: when is 'statistically significant' clinically useful? Breast Cancer Res Treat 1998;52:305–319.

Henson DE, Fielding P, Grignon DJ, Page DL, Hammond ME, Nash G, Pettigrew NM, Gorstein F, Hutter RV: College of American Pathologists Conference XXVI on clinical relevance of prognostic markers in solid tumors. Arch Pathol Lab Med 1995;19:1109–1112.

Higuchi R, Fockler C, Dollinger G, Watson R: Kinetic PCR: real time monitoring of DNA amplification reactions. Biotech 1993;11:1026–1030.

Hynes NE: Amplification and overexpression of the erbB-2 gene in human tumors: its involvement in tumor development, significance as a prognostic factor, and potential as a target for cancer therapy. Semin Cancer Biol 1993;4:19–26.

Hynes NE, Stern DF: The biology of erbB-2/neu/HER-2 and its role in cancer. Biochim Biophys Acta Rev Cancer 1994;1198:165–184.

Jacobs TW, Gown AM, Yaziji H, Barnes MJ, Schnitt SJ: HER-2/neu protein expression in breast cancer evaluated by immunohistochemistry. Am J Clin Pathol 2000;113:251–256.

Jacobs TW, Gown AM, Yaziji H, Barnes MJ, Schnitt SJ: Comparison of fluorescence in-situ hybridization and immunohistochemistry for the evaluation of HER-2/neu in breast cancer. J Clin Oncol 1999a;17:1974–1982.

Jacobs TW, Gown AM, Yaziji H, Barnes MJ, Schnitt SJ: Specificity of HercepTest in determining HER-2/neu status of breast cancers using the United States Food and Drug Administration-approved scoring system. J Clin Oncol 1999b;17:1983–1987.

Jacobs TW, Prioleau JE, Stillman IE, Schnitt SJ: Loss of tumor marker-immunostaining intensity on stored paraffin slides of breast cancer. J Natl Cancer Inst 1996;88:1054–1059.

Jiminez RE, Wallis, T, Tabasczka P, Visscher DW: Determination of Her-2/Neu status in breast carcinoma: a comparative analysis of immunohistochemistry and fluorescence in situ hybridization. Mod Pathol 2000;13:37–45.

Kay EW, Walsh CJ, Cassidy M, Curran B, Leader M: C-erbB-2 immunostaining: problems with interpretation. J Clin Pathol 1994;47:816–822.

Lehmann U, Glockner S, Kleeberger W, von Wasielewski HF, Kreipe H: Detection of gene amplification in archival breast cancer specimens by laser-assisted microdissection and quantitative real-time polymerase chain reaction. Am J Pathol 2000;156:1855–1864.

Maia DM: Immunohistochemical assays for HER2 overexpression. J Clin Oncol 1999;17:1650.

Mass RD, Sanders C, Charlene K, Johnson L, Everett T, Anderson S: The concordance between the clinical trials assay (CTA) and fluorescence in situ hybridisation (FISH) in the Herceptin pivotal trials. Proc Am Soc Clin Oncol 2000; 19:75A.

McGuire WL: Breast cancer prognostic factors: evaluation guidelines. J Natl Cancer Inst 1991; 83:1–9.

Ménard S, Fortis S, Castiglioni F, Agresti R, Balsari A: HER2 as a prognostic factor in breast cancer. Oncology 2001;61(suppl 2):67–72.

Nelson NJ: Common techniques used to detect HER2. J Natl Cancer Inst 2000;92:293–294.
Norton L, Slamon D, Leyland-Jones B, Wolter J, Fleming T, Eirmann W, Baselga J, Mendelsohn J, Bajamonde A, Ash M, Shak S: Overall survival (OS) advantage to Herceptin (H) in HER2-overexpressing (HER2+) metastatic breast cancer (MBC). Proc Am Soc Clin Oncol 1999;18:127A.
Okuyama N, Hatano Y, Park Y, Shimatani S, Sasamoto S, Katou N, Takagi K, Yamazaki S, Inoue A, Hemmi H, Shimatake H, Yanagida M, Miura M: Quantitation of c-erbB-2 gene amplification in breast cancer tissue by competitive PCR. Tumour Biol 1999;20:153–161.
O'Malley FP, Parkes R, Hanna W, et al: A Canadian interlaboratory concordance study of HER2/neu assessment by immunohistochemistry and FISH. Mod Pathol 2001;14:33A.
Paik S, Bryant J, Park C, Fisher B, Tan-Chiu E, Hyams D, Fisher ER, Lippman ME, Wickerham DL, Wolmark N: Erb-B2 and response to doxorubicin in patients with axillary lymph node-positive, hormone-receptor-negative breast cancer. J Natl Cancer Inst 1998;90:1361–1370.
Pauletti G, Godolphin W, Press MF, Slamon DJ: Detection and quantitation of HER-2/neu gene amplification in human breast cancer archival material using fluorescence in situ hybridization. Oncogene 1996;13:63–72.
Penault-Llorca F, Adelaide J, Houvenaeghel G, Hassoun J, Birnbaun D, Jacquemier J: Optimization of immunohistochemical detection of ERBB" in human breast cancer: impact of fixation. J Pathol 1994;173:65–75.
Persons DL, Bui MM, Lowery MC, Mark HF, Yung JF, Birkmeier JM, Wong EY, Yang SJ, Masood S: Fluorescence in situ hybridization (FISH) for detection of HER-2/neu amplification in breast cancer: a multicenter portability study. Ann Clin Lab Sci 2000;30:41–48.
Piccart M, Awada A, Hamilton A: Integration of new therapies into management of metastatic breast cancer: a focus on chemotherapy, treatment selection through use of molecular markers, and newly developed biologic therapies in late clinical development. Am Soc Clin Oncol 1999;35th Annual Meeting, May 15–18, Atlanta. Educational Book 526–539.
Piccart M, Lohrisch C, Di Leo A, Larsimont D: The predictive value of HER2 in breast cancer. Oncology 2001;61(suppl 2):73–82.
Press MF, Hung G, Godolphin W, Slamon DJ: Sensitivity of HER2/neu antibodies in archival tissue samples: potential source of error in immunohistochemical studies of oncogene expression. Cancer Res 1994;54:2771–2777.
Ratcliffe N, Wells W, Wheeler K, Memoli V: The combination of in situ hybridization and immunohistochemical analysis: an evaluation of HER2/neu expression in paraffin-embedded breast carcinomas and adjacent normal-appearing breast epithelium. Mod Pathol 1997; 10:1247–1252.
Roche PC, Ingle JN: Increased HER2 with U.S. Food and Drug Administration-approved antibody. J Clin Oncol 1999;17:434.
Ross JS, Fletcher JA: The HER-2/neu oncogene in breast cancer: prognostic factor, predictive factor, and target for therapy. Stem Cells 1998;16: 413–428.
Slamon DJ, Clark GM, Wong SG, Levin WJ, Ullrich A, McGuire WL: Human breast cancer: correlation of relapse and survival with amplification of the HER-2/neu oncogene. Science 1987;235:177–182.
Slamon DJ, Godolphin W, Jones LA, Holt JA, Wong SG, Keith DE, Levin WJ, Stuart SG, Udove J, Ullrich A: Studies of the HER-2/neu proto-oncogene in human breast and ovarian cancer. Science 1989;244:707–712.
Slamon D, Leyland-Jones B, Shak S, Paton V, Bajamonde A, Fleming T, Eiermann W, Wolter J, Baselga J, Norton L: Addition of Herceptin™ (humanized anti-HER2 antibody) to first-line chemotherapy for HER2 overexpressing metastatic breast cancer (HER2+/MBC) markedly increases anticancer activity: a randomized, multinational controlled phase III trial. Proc Am Soc Clin Oncol 1998;17:98A.
Slamon DJ, Leyland-Jones B, Shak S, Fuchs H, Paton V, Bajamonde A, Fleming T, Eiermann W, Wolter J, Pegram M, Baselga J, Norton L: Use of chemotherapy plus a monoclonal antibody against HER2 for metastatic breast cancer that overexpresses HER2. N Engl J Med 2001;344:783–792.
Tandon AK, Clark GM, Chamness GC, Ullrich A, McGuire WL: HER-2/neu oncogene protein and prognosis in breast cancer. J Clin Oncol 1989;7:1120–1128.
Thor AD, Schwartz LH, Koerner FC, Edgerton SM, Skates SJ, Yin S, McKenzie SJ, Panicali DL, Marks PJ, Fingert AJ, et al: Analysis of c-erbB-2 expression in breast carcinomas with clinical follow-up. Cancer Res 1989;49:7147–7152.
Thor AD, Berry DA, Budman DR, Muss HB, Kute T, Henderson IC, Barcos M, Cirrincione C, Edgerton S, Allred C, Norton L, Liu ET: Erb-B2, p53 and efficacy of adjuvant therapy in lymph node-positive breast cancer. J Natl Cancer Inst 1998;90:1346–1360.
Vogel CL, Cobleigh M, Tripathy D, Harris L, Fehrenbacher L, Slamon D, Ash M, Novotny W, Stewart S, Shak S: First-line, non-hormonal treatment of women with HER2 overexpressing metastatic breast cancer with Herceptin (trastuzumab, humanized anti-HER2 antibody). Proc Am Soc Clin Oncol 2000;19:71A.
Vogel CL, Cobleigh MA, Tripathy D, Gutheil JC, Harris LN, Fehrenbacher L, Slamon DJ, Murphy M, Novotny WF, Burchmore M, Shak S, Stewart SJ: First-line Herceptin® monotherapy in metastatic breast cancer. Oncology 2001; 61(suppl 2):37–42.
Vona G, Caldini A, Sestini R, Rapi S, Bianchi S, Fanelli A, Pazzagli M, Orlando C: The c-erbB-2 oncogene amplification by competitive PCR in aneuploid cell clones flow sorted from breast cancer samples. Clin Chem Lab Med 1999;37: 649–654.
Youngson BJ, Anelli A, Van Zee KJ, Borgen PI, Norton L, Rosen PP: Microdissection and molecular genetic analysis of HER2/neu in breast carcinoma. Am J Surg Pathol 1995:19:1354–1368.

Oncology

Oncology 2001;61(suppl 2):31–36

Dose Scheduling – Herceptin®

Brian Leyland-Jones

Department of Oncology, McGill University, Montreal, Que., Canada

Key Words
Herceptin® · Metastatic breast cancer · Combination therapy · Single agent · Subcutaneous · Pharmacokinetics · 3-weekly

Abstract
Preclinical and phase I/II studies of Herceptin® demonstrated a dose-related, non-linear pharmacokinetic profile. The results of a dose-finding study supported a regimen comprising an initial intravenous (i.v.) dose of 4 mg/kg with subsequent weekly doses of 2 mg/kg. However, pharmacokinetic and safety data suggested that increased dose and reduced frequency of Herceptin administration are feasible. In addition, evidence shows that Herceptin plus paclitaxel has additive antitumor efficacy in vitro, and this regimen produces significant clinical benefits. These observations form the rationale for conducting a phase I/II trial of Herceptin (8 mg/kg initial dose, 6 mg/kg maintenance dose) plus paclitaxel, both given 3-weekly. Preliminary results are promising, with serum trough Herceptin concentrations being similar and AUC being greater than those observed with weekly Herceptin plus 3-weekly paclitaxel. Two further trials are proposed: 3-weekly Herceptin as first-line monotherapy of metastatic breast cancer; and 3-weekly Herceptin with the oral 5-fluorouracil derivative, Xeloda® (capecitabine). Subcutaneous (s.c.) administration of Herceptin would further simplify administration and studies are also underway to clinically evaluate s.c. administration of Herceptin in combination with paclitaxel. With the recent development of oral taxanes, it is predicted that combinations including an oral taxane, Xeloda and either 3-weekly or possibly s.c. Herceptin may become future therapies for breast cancer patients.

Introduction

Metastatic breast cancer continues to be a devastating and mostly incurable disease. However, recent years have seen the rapid development of a number of novel therapies that offer meaningful palliation and prolongation of survival for some patients [de Valeriola et al. 1997; Miller and Sledge 1999]. Among the new anticancer agents contributing to improved outcomes in metastatic breast cancer is the biological anticancer agent, Herceptin® (trastuzumab) [Carter et al. 1992; Cobleigh et al. 1999; Slamon et al. 2001]. Treatment advances have also been made by modulating drug administration schedules and routes (e.g., the introduction of i.v. or intra-arterial administration) [Terwogt et al. 1999], changing drug formulation (e.g., by encapsulating chemotherapeutic drugs in liposomes or binding them to polymers) [Terwogt et al. 1999], and introducing new drug combinations (e.g., Herceptin plus taxanes) [Slamon et al. 2001]. Both alone and combined, these strategies are proving successful in improving cancer survival and cure rates [Ferrante et al. 1999; Greco and Hainsworth 1999; Miller and Sledge 1999; Rich 1999].

New drug development requires extensive and thorough optimization of drug formulation, route of administration and selection of combination therapy [de Valerio-

KARGER
Fax + 41 61 306 12 34
E-Mail karger@karger.ch
www.karger.com

0030–2414/01/0616–0031$17.50/0

Accessible online at:
www.karger.com/journals/ocl

B. Leyland-Jones, MD
Department of Oncology, McGill University
Suite 701, 3655 Drummond Avenue
Montreal, H3G 1Y6 (Canada)
Tel. +1 514 398 8986, Fax +1 514 398 6769, E-Mail leylandj@med.mcgill.ca

la et al. 1997; Masson et al. 1997; Terwogt et al. 1999]. The pharmacology and pharmacokinetics of new drugs must also be well characterized [Masson et al. 1997; Terwogt et al. 1999]. Drug bioavailability, which determines the optimal formulation, is controlled by physicochemical properties. Likewise, drug distribution and serum concentration, which determine the optimal schedule and route of administration, are controlled by pharmacokinetics. In addition to drug physicochemical and pharmacokinetic properties, knowledge of the mechanism of action and pharmacodynamics between the drug and its target is also critically important.

Herceptin is a humanized monoclonal antibody directed against the extracellular domain (ECD) of the human epidermal growth factor receptor-2 (HER2) [Carter et al. 1992]. The HER2 receptor is overexpressed in 20 to 30% of breast cancers [Hynes and Stern 1994] and predicts for a poor clinical outcome [for a review, see Ross and Fletcher 1998]. Herceptin is approved for the treatment of HER2-positive metastatic breast cancer as an initial dose of 4 mg/kg i.v. over 90 min followed by weekly doses of 2 mg/kg i.v. over 30 min until disease progression, either alone or in combination with taxanes [Goldenberg 1999]. This dose schedule was established on the basis of its pharmacokinetics, tolerability and consideration of the minimum effective serum concentration [Baselga et al. 1996; Carter et al. 1992; Pegram et al. 1998; Tokuda et al. 1996].

Clinical trials are currently being conducted or are planned to evaluate alternative dose schedules and routes of administration for Herceptin. This paper reviews the pharmacokinetics of Herceptin in relation to dose scheduling and describes how this knowledge is leading to trials to evaluate Herceptin in 3-weekly schedules, both alone and in combination with chemotherapeutic agents. A number of studies to assess the clinical relevance of s.c. administration of Herceptin are also described.

Preclinical Data

The humanized murine anti-HER2 monoclonal antibody (MAb) Herceptin, has an in vitro binding affinity for the HER2 ECD 3-fold that of 4D5, the precursor to Herceptin (Kd = 0.1 n*M*) [Carter et al. 1992]. Herceptin was also shown to be cytostatic and to mediate antibody-dependent cellular cytotoxicity against HER2-positive cells in these and other in vitro studies [Carter et al. 1992; Hotaling et al. 1996]. Preclinical pharmacokinetic studies of Herceptin using animal models have revealed slow serum clearance (<0.7 ml/kg/h) and a long terminal half-life (at least one week) (data on file, F. Hoffmann-La Roche Ltd). Maximal tumor growth inhibition was associated with antibody concentrations of between 1 and 23 µg/ml (data on file, F. Hoffmann-La Roche Ltd). Thus, a minimum serum trough concentration of 10 µg/ml was considered necessary for a therapeutic response in humans and was therefore targeted in clinical studies [Carter et al. 1992; Tokuda et al. 1996].

Clinical Studies

The tolerability of Herceptin was evaluated in two small phase I trials of multiple weekly doses of i.v. Herceptin (10 to 500 mg) alone (n = 17) or in combination with cisplatin i.v. (100 mg/m^2) (n = 15) administered on a four-weekly dose schedule. The maximum tolerated dose was not reached in either study and concomitant administration of cisplatin did not influence the pharmacokinetic profile of Herceptin (data on file, F. Hoffmann-La Roche Ltd). Two larger phase II studies examined Herceptin 250 mg i.v. followed by weekly doses of 100 mg i.v. until disease progression with (n = 46) or without (n = 39) cisplatin 75 mg/m^2 every four weeks [Baselga et al. 1996; Pegram et al. 1998]. In the single-agent trial, >90% of patients had Herceptin trough levels above the target level of 10 µg/ml and the mean serum half-life of Herceptin was 8.3 days [Baselga et al. 1996]. In the Herceptin plus cisplatin trial, the mean trough and peak Herceptin concentrations were approximately 79 µg/ml and 123 µg/ml, respectively, and the mean half-life was 5.8 days [Pegram et al. 1998].

Overall, the phase I and II trials showed that the terminal half-life of Herceptin increased from 1.1 to 23 days and the clearance decreased from 38.0 to 4.1 ml/day, with increasing doses from 10 to 500 mg (table 1). This dose-related, non-linear pharmacokinetic profile is consistent with saturation of a specific receptor-mediated clearance mechanism. Importantly, the targeted minimum trough concentration of 10 µg/ml was achieved in the majority of patients receiving the 100 mg weekly dose, and this was identified as the weekly dose likely to achieve clinical efficacy. In order to achieve the targeted serum concentration more quickly, a loading dose (250 mg) was introduced in a phase II trial. However, further analyses suggested that clinical efficacy may be effected more consistently by adjusting the dose by body weight. A trend towards clinical response in patients receiving 1.6 to 1.9 mg/kg was identified and lent support to a regimen comprising an initial dose of 4 mg/kg with subsequent weekly doses of 2 mg/kg. This regimen was therefore used in two pivotal

Table 1. Pharmacokinetics in phase I and II trials using various doses of Herceptin

Dose, mg/ regimen	Dose mg/kg	Patients	Cmax mg/ml	Half-life days	Clearance ml/day/kg
10/sd	0.163 ± 0.0006	3	3.0 ± 0.064	1.1 ± 0.26	38.0 ± 7.2
50/sd	0.787 ± 0.124	3	19.0 ± 8.6	2.8 ± 0.64	13.0 ± 1.1
100/sd	1.433 ± 0.451	3	29.0 ± 7.4	3.3 ± 0.28	12.0 ± 4.2
250/sd	3.7 ± 1.02	4	93.0 ± 23.0	13.0 ± 11.0	6.1 ± 1.9
500/sd	7.7 ± 1.31	3	170.0	23.0 ± 1.9	4.1
100/md	1.55 ± 0.30	84	116.0 ± 62.0	9.02 ± 9.76	6.26 ± 7.44

clinical trials of Herceptin therapy in patients with metastatic HER2-positive breast cancer.

The pivotal trials of Herceptin demonstrated a mean terminal half-life of 6 to 10 days and a mean trough serum Herceptin concentration in the range of 50 to 55 μg/ml. The computed steady state concentrations were 50 to 55 μg/ml, and steady state was achieved at 12 to 32 weeks. Furthermore, Herceptin was well tolerated at these doses [Slamon et al. 2001]. While the available pharmacokinetic and tolerability data support the current Herceptin dose and schedule, clinical evidence of increasing half-life with increasing dose and complex clearance mechanisms leading to a long terminal half-life lend support to a reduction in frequency of administration. Extending the time between Herceptin doses is attractive, particularly in the adjuvant setting where the burden of therapy becomes more of an issue.

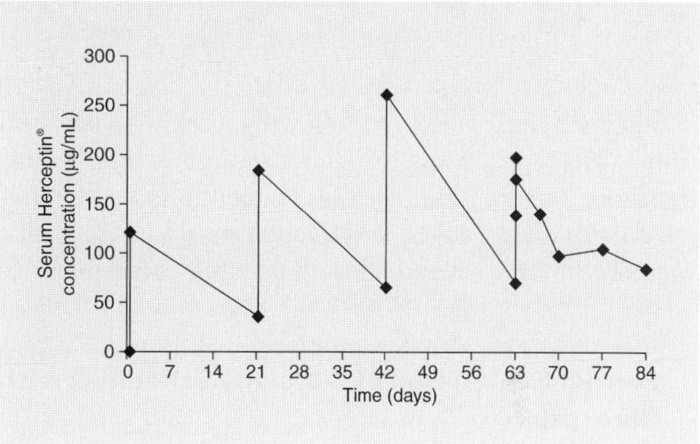

Fig. 1. Serum Herceptin concentration in a patient treated with 3-weekly Herceptin.

Phase I/II Study of 3-Weekly Herceptin Plus Paclitaxel

Preclinical studies showed additive tumor growth inhibition when Herceptin is combined with paclitaxel [Pegram et al. 1999]. Furthermore, a large randomized controlled phase III trial provided clear clinical evidence that adding Herceptin to paclitaxel as first-line therapy for advanced disease provides substantial clinical benefits that include an increased survival rate [Slamon et al. 2001].

As is the case with many anticancer agents, paclitaxel is administered according to a 3-weekly regimen. The pharmacokinetic and tolerability data indicate that higher doses of Herceptin are likely to be well tolerated and could be administered at longer intervals such as once every 3 weeks. A 3-weekly regimen of Herceptin plus paclitaxel is an attractive proposition and would have particular relevance to patients receiving adjuvant therapy.

A phase I/II trial of Herceptin plus paclitaxel, both given 3-weekly, in women with HER2-positive metastatic breast cancer is currently ongoing. The primary aim of this trial is to characterize the pharmacokinetic profile of a Herceptin 6 mg/kg dose by i.v. administration every 3 weeks following an initial dose of 8 mg/kg. The secondary trial objective is to evaluate the safety and tolerability of 3-weekly Herceptin plus paclitaxel. Simulation of the proposed treatment regimen of 3-weekly Herceptin has indicated that the trough concentrations will be in the range of 40 to 50 μg/ml, similar to that observed in the pivotal trials.

Significantly, the preliminary data from this study indicate that the 3-weekly dosing schedule for Herceptin is compatible with maintenance of biologically active levels of the drug. Herceptin levels observed in a typical patient following 3-weekly administration in combination with paclitaxel are shown in figure 1. The measured trough levels are approximately 40, 55 and 60 μg/ml, con-

Table 2. Combination index values for Herceptin interactions with other chemotherapy agents

Drug	Combination index	p value	Interaction
Cisplatin	0.048	0.003	synergism
Thiotepa	0.67	0.0008	synergism
Etoposide	0.54	0.0003	synergism
Doxorubicin	1.16	0.13	addition
Paclitaxel	0.91	0.21	addition
Methotrexate	1.15	0.28	addition
Vinblastine	1.09	0.26	addition
5-fluorouracil	2.87	0.0001	antagonism

sistent with those observed following weekly administration of Herceptin using the standard dose schedule. Furthermore, the data indicate that Herceptin is well tolerated at these higher doses, and the pharmacokinetic profile suggests that the 3-weekly dosing schedule is feasible.

Further Exploration of 3-Weekly Schedules with Herceptin

The encouraging data from the phase I/II study of 3-weekly Herceptin plus paclitaxel have prompted the design of two further trials to evaluate 3-weekly schedules containing Herceptin. The first of these aims to assess the response rate and tolerability of Herceptin as a single agent in first-line treatment of metastatic breast cancer. In this study, which is projected to include 80 HER2-positive patients, 3-weekly Herceptin will be administered as an 8-mg/kg initial dose followed by a maintenance dose of 6 mg/kg.

The second trial will address combination therapy comprising Herceptin plus the 5-fluorouracil derivative, Xeloda® (capecitabine). Xeloda is a selectively tumor-activated oral fluoropyrimidine carbamate with activity against a variety of solid tumors including breast and colon cancer [Blum 1999]. In a series of in vitro and in vivo experiments, Pegram and coworkers [1999] examined the interactions between clinically relevant concentrations of Herceptin and a range of cytotoxic drugs using a multiple drug effect/combination index (CI) isobologram analysis (table 2). Synergistic activity against HER2-overexpressing tumor cells was observed with cisplatin, thiotepa, and etoposide, and additive effects were observed with doxorubicin, paclitaxel, methotrexate and vinblastine. Although the authors reported an antagonistic interaction between Herceptin and 5-fluorouracil, it must be noted that the pharmacodynamic definition of antagonism used in their analysis was relatively strict. Antagonism was defined as a response that was less than the additive effects of both drugs administered separately. Thus, if the combination of two drugs with separate efficacies of 30 and 40% yields a 60% effect, the interaction was defined as antagonistic. In clinical practice, a 60% rate would be regarded favorably.

Anecdotal responses have been observed with the Herceptin plus Xeloda combination, and preliminary results from a European trial indicate that responses can be obtained in up to 50% of extensively pretreated patients [Bangemann et al. 2000]. Thus, a number of trials are already underway to assess the tolerability and efficacy of combined Xeloda therapies in breast cancer [Elza-Brown et al. 2000; Venturini et al. 2000]. A phase II randomized study to evaluate the response rate and tolerability of Herceptin plus Xeloda is at the planning stage. Patients will receive 3-weekly Herceptin and 40 patients will be recruited.

Orally active chemotherapy is a particularly attractive option for patients whose access to hospital is limited by financial considerations, long journeys or for patients who are reluctant to receive injections [Marty et al. 1999]. With the recent development of oral taxanes [Nicoletti et al. 2000; Polizzi et al. 2000], it is predicted that combinations including an oral taxane, the oral chemotherapeutic agent, Xeloda, and either 3-weekly Herceptin, or possibly s.c. Herceptin may become new therapeutic options in metastatic breast cancer. Such combined therapies are anticipated to reduce the need for in-patient therapy. Furthermore, should s.c. administration of Herceptin prove feasible, as discussed below, therapy could be provided to breast cancer patients in an entirely out-patient setting.

Subcutaneous Administration of Herceptin

Less invasive drug administration routes are preferred by patients, provided that efficacy is not compromised [Liu et al 1997]. Moreover, i.v. administration is cited by patients as a source of discomfort [Coates et al. 1983]. These findings mean that further research into optimal administration route as well as frequency of dosing is warranted. Subcutaneous administration of Herceptin would be a simple, potentially self-administered alternative to the current practice and would be a particularly attractive option for women treated in the adjuvant setting. Self-dosing also potentially eliminates administration and nursing costs, which are known to incur a large component of the total cost of i.v. chemotherapy [Marty et al. 1999].

Preclinical data relating to the s.c. administration of Herceptin has been obtained from studies in monkeys. Four monkeys received 2 mg/kg s.c. injection and four received a 2-mg/kg i.v. injection. In this study, the bioavailability of Herceptin following s.c. administration was determined to be 54% [data on file, Genentech, Inc.]. In addition, there was no evidence of toxicity and antibody formation did not occur. These promising results have formed the basis of a clinical evaluation of s.c. administration of Herceptin. In this study, patients will receive paclitaxel in combination with Herceptin given either weekly or twice weekly for 22 weeks, or until disease progression. Herceptin therapy will be continued in responding patients until disease progression or week 48. The study will be preceded by a single-dose study, in which s.c. Herceptin monotherapy will be administered to 16 patients, followed by a 2-week washout period. In this way, it is anticipated that the study will yield useful data pertaining to the pharmacokinetics, biological efficacy and tolerability of s.c. Herceptin.

The s.c. injection will be given into the anterior abdominal wall using a 25-gauge needle. The increased frequency of administration compared with that for i.v. administration reflects volume constraints. The reconstituted s.c. injection vial will contain 4.4 ml at a Herceptin concentration of 102 mg/ml. The average injection volume for a 2-mg/kg dose will therefore be approximately 1.4 ml for an average 70-kg person. It is anticipated that this injection volume, although quite large, will be well tolerated.

Conclusions

In summary, clinical studies with Herceptin have demonstrated that a regimen comprising an initial dose of 4 mg/kg and weekly administration of 2 mg/kg is associated with significant clinical benefit and is well tolerated. Pharmacokinetic data also suggest that higher doses of Herceptin are likely to be associated with longer half-life and slower clearance and well tolerated. Thus, higher Herceptin doses could be administered less frequently, while still maintaining serum drug levels associated with clinical benefit. The pharmacokinetics of Herceptin are such that dose intervals of up to 3 weeks are feasible, which would facilitate a more convenient regimen for combination therapies and would be attractive to patients, especially in the adjuvant setting. Preliminary results of a phase I/II study of 3-weekly Herceptin (8 mg/kg initial dose, 6 mg/kg maintenance dose) in combination with paclitaxel suggest that biologically active levels of Herceptin are maintained and that the combination is well tolerated. Two further studies are under consideration: a trial of first-line, 3-weekly, single-agent Herceptin therapy for metastatic breast cancer, and a trial of Herceptin 3-weekly in combination with the oral 5-fluorouracil derivative, Xeloda. Clinical evaluation of s.c. administration of Herceptin is also planned. A reduced frequency of administration of Herceptin will confer significant advantages compared with the existing regimen, particularly in patients receiving Herceptin adjuvant therapy. The administration of Herceptin by s.c. injection would further reduce in-patient treatment time. The results of these clinical trials are eagerly awaited.

References

Bangemann N, Kuhle A, Ebert A, Bühler H, Schaller G: Capecitabine combined with trastuzumab in the therapy of intensively pretreated HER2-overexpressing metastatic breast cancer (MBC). Ann Oncol 2000;11(suppl 4):143(abstract 653P).

Baselga J, Tripathy D, Mendelsohn J, Baughman S, Benz CC, Dantis L, Sklarin NT, Seidman AD, Hudis CA, Moore J, Rosen P, Twaddell T, Henderson IC, Norton L: Phase II study of weekly intravenous recombinant humanized anti-p185^{HER2} monoclonal antibody in patients with HER2/*neu*-overexpressing metastatic breast cancer. J Clin Oncol 1996;14:737–744.

Blum JL: Xeloda in the treatment of metastatic breast cancer. Oncology 1999;57(suppl 1):16–20.

Carter P, Presta L, Gorman CM, Ridgway JBB, Henner D, Wong WLT, Rowland AM, Kotts C, Carver ME, Shephard HM: Humanization of an anti-p185HER2 antibody for human cancer therapy. Proc Natl Acad Sci USA 1992;89:4285–4289.

Coates A, Abraham S, Kaye SB, Sowerbutts T, Frewin C, Fox RM, Tattersall MH: On the receiving end – patient perceptions of the side effects of cancer chemotherapy. Eur J Cancer Clin Oncol 1983;19:203–208.

Cobleigh MA, Vogel CL, Tripathy D, Robert NJ, Scholl S, Fehrenbacher L, Wolter JM, Paton V, Shak S, Lieberman G, Slamon DJ: Multinational study of the efficacy and safety of humanized anti-HER2 monoclonal antibody in women who have HER2-overexpressing metastatic breast cancer that has progressed after chemotherapy for metastatic disease. J Clin Oncol 1999;17:2639–2648.

de Valeriola D, Awada A, Roy J-A, DiLeo A, Biganzoli L, Piccart M: Breast cancer therapies in development: a review of their pharmacology and clinical potential. Drugs 1997;54:385–413.

Elza-Brown K, Dees EC, Wolff AC, Carducci MA, Donehower RC: A phase I study of capecitabine and weekly paclitaxel in advanced solid tumors. Proc Am Soc Clin Oncol 2000;19:237A.

Ferrante K, Winograd B, Canetta R: Promising new developments in cancer chemotherapy. Cancer Chemother Pharmacol 1999;43:S61–S68.

Oncology 2001;61(suppl 2):31–36

Goldenberg MM: Trastuzumab, a recombinant DNA-derived humanized monoclonal antibody, a novel agent for the treatment of metastatic breast cancer. Clin Ther 1999;21:309–318.

Greco FA, Hainsworth JD: Paclitaxel-based therapy in non-small-cell lung cancer: improved third generation chemotherapy. Ann Oncol 1999;10(suppl 5):S63–S67.

Hotaling TE, Reitz B, Wolfgang-Kimball D, et al: The humanized anti-HER2 antibody rhuMAb HER2 mediates antibody dependent cell-mediated cytotoxicity via FcγRIII. Proc Annu Meet Am Assoc Cancer Res 1996;37:471(abstract).

Hynes NE, Stern DF: The biology of *erbB-2/neu/HER-2* and its role in cancer. Biochim Biophys Acta 1994;1198:165–184.

Liu G, Franssen E, Fitch MI, Warner E: Patient preferences for oral versus intravenous palliative chemotherapy. J Clin Oncol 1997;15:110–115.

Marty M, Espie M, Cottu PH, Cuvier C, Lerebours F: Optimizing chemotherapy for patients with advanced breast cancer. Oncology 1999;57 (suppl 1):21–26.

Masson E, Zamboni WC: Pharmacokinetic optimisation of cancer chemotherapy: effects on outcomes. Clin Pharmacokinet 1997;32:324–343.

Miller KD, Sledge GW Jr: Taxanes in the treatment of breast cancer: a prodigy comes of age. Cancer Invest 1999;17:121–136.

Nicoletti MI, Colombo T, Rossi C, Monardo C, Stura S, Zucchetti M, Riva A, Morazzoni P, Donati MB, Bombardelli E, D'Incalci M, Giavazzi R: IDN5109, a taxane with oral bioavailability and potent antitumor activity. Cancer Res 2000;60:842–846.

Pegram M, Hsu S, Lewis G, Pietras R, Beryt M, Sliwkowski M, Coombs D, Baly D, Kabbinavar F, Slamon D: Inhibitory effects of combinations of HER-2/neu antibody and chemotherapeutic agents used for treatment of human breast cancers. Oncogene 1999;18:2241–2251.

Pegram MD, Lipton A, Hayes DF, Weber BL, Baselga JM, Tripathy D, Baly D, Baughman SA, Twaddell T, Glaspy JA, Slamon DJ: Phase II study of receptor-enhanced chemosensitivity using recombinant humanized anti-p185^{HER2} monoclonal antibody plus cisplatin in patients with HER-2/*neu*-overexpressing metastatic breast cancer refractory to chemotherapy treatment. J Clin Oncol 1998;16:2659-2671.

Polizzi D, Pratesi G, Monestiroli S, Tortoreto M, Zunino F, Bombardelli E, Riva A, Morazzoni P, Colombo T, D'Incalci M, Zucchetti M: Oral efficacy and bioavailability of a novel taxane. Clin Cancer Res 2000;6:2070–2074.

Rich TA: Infusional chemoradiation for rectal and anal cancers. Oncology (Huntingt) 1999;3 (suppl 5):131–134 .

Ross JS, Fletcher JA: The HER-2/*neu* oncogene in breast cancer: prognostic factor, predictive factor, and target for therapy. Stem Cells 1998;16: 413–428.

Slamon DJ, Leyland-Jones B, Shak S, Fuchs H, Paton V, Bajamonde A, Fleming T, Eiermann W, Wolter J, Pegram M, Baselga J, Norton L: Use of chemotherapy plus a monoclonal antibody against HER2 for metastatic breast cancer that overexpresses HER2. N Engl J Med 2001;344:783–792.

Terwogt JMM, Schellens JHM, ten Bokkel Huinink WW, Beijnen JH: Clinical pharmacology of anticancer agents in relation to formulations and administration routes. Cancer Treat Rev 1999;25:83–101.

Tokuda Y, Ohnishi Y, Shimamura K, Iwasawa M, Yoshimura M, Ueyama Y, Tamaoki N, Tajima T, Mitomi T: In vitro and in vivo anti-tumour effects of a humanised monoclonal antibody against c-erbB-2 product. Br J Cancer 1996;73: 1362–1365.

Venturini M, Del Mastro L, Merlano M, Angiolini C, Straneo M, tolino G, Garrone O, Bergaglio M, Lambniase A, Bertelli G, Signorini A, Rosso R: Dose finding study of capecitabine in combination with docetaxel and epirubicin in prior untreated advanced breast cancer patients. Proc Am Soc Clin Oncol 2000;19:108A.

Oncology

Oncology 2001;61(suppl 2):37–42

First-Line Herceptin® Monotherapy in Metastatic Breast Cancer

Charles L. Vogel[a] Melody A. Cobleigh[b] Debu Tripathy[c] John C. Gutheil[d] Lyndsay N. Harris[e] Louis Fehrenbacher[f] Dennis J. Slamon[g] Maureen Murphy[h] William F. Novotny[h] Michael Burchmore[h] Steven Shak[h] Stanford J. Stewart[h]

[a]University of Miami School of Medicine, Comprehensive Cancer Research Group, Inc., and Columbia Cancer Research Network of Florida, Miami, Fla., [b]Rush-Presbytarian-St Luke's Medical Center, Chicago, Ill., [c]UCSF/Mount Zion Cancer Center, San Francisco, Calif., [d]Vical, Inc., San Diego, Calif., [e]Dana Farber Cancer Institute, Boston, Mass., [f]Kaiser Permanante, Vallejo, Calif., [g]UCLA School of Medicine, Los Angeles, Calif., [h]Genentech, Inc., South San Francisco, Calif., USA

Key Words

First-line therapy · FISH · HER2 positive · Herceptin® · IHC 3+ · Metastatic breast cancer · Monotherapy

Abstract

The pivotal phase II and III Herceptin® trials proved the efficacy and safety of second- or third-line single-agent Herceptin and first-line Herceptin in combination with chemotherapy, respectively. In the current trial, 114 patients were randomized to one of two dose groups of first-line Herceptin monotherapy: standard dose of 4 mg/kg initial dose followed by 2 mg/kg intravenous (i.v.) weekly; or high dose of 8 mg/kg initial dose followed by 4 mg/kg i.v. weekly. The regimen was generally well tolerated. A similar incidence of adverse events was demonstrated in the two dose groups with the possible exception of acute infusion-related events such as fever and chills as well as rash and dyspnea, which appear to be more prevalent in the higher dose group. The overall response rate was 26% and response rates were similar between the two dose groups (24% for the standard Herceptin dose group and 28% for the high Herceptin dose group). Subgroup analysis determined a higher response rate in IHC 3+ patients (35%) and FISH-positive patients (41%). When women with stable disease for ≥6 months were included with responders, the clinical benefit rate in IHC 3+ patients was 47%. Median survival was 24.4 months, which is comparable with the survival rate seen in the pivotal phase III combination trial (25 months). Therefore, single-agent Herceptin is an important new option for the first-line treatment of HER2-positive metastatic breast cancer patients.

Introduction

Despite recent advances in therapy for breast cancer, more than 43,000 women in the USA die of metastatic breast cancer each year [Hortobagyi 1998; Landis et al. 1999]. Recently, investigators have evaluated the role of several molecular factors thought to be involved in tumor cell proliferation in order to identify potential targets for novel therapies. The human epidermal growth factor-2 (HER2) is one such factor that has been shown to be

KARGER

Fax + 41 61 306 12 34
E-Mail karger@karger.ch
www.karger.com

0030–2414/01/0616–0037$17.50/0

Accessible online at:
www.karger.com/journals/ocl

Prof. Charles Vogel
South Point Medical Center
600 South Pine Island Rd Ste 104
Plantation, FL 33324 (USA)
Tel. +1 954 473 6776, Fax +1 954 473 4552

involved in tumorigenicity [Benz et al. 1992; Di Fiore et al. 1987a, b; Hudziak et al. 1987]. As a consequence, a humanized anti-HER2 monoclonal antibody, Herceptin®, was rationally developed to target HER2-overexpressing breast tumors [Carter et al. 1992].

Preclinical data have demonstrated that Herceptin exerts potent antiproliferative/antitumor activity in ovarian and breast cancer cell lines and in human breast cancer xenograft models [Baselga et al. 1998; Carter et al. 1992; Lewis et al. 1993; Pegram et al. 1992, 1997, 1999]. Based on these data and preclinical pharamacokinetic and favorable toxicology studies, a clinical trial program of Herceptin in small numbers of patients was initiated. Two open-label, phase I dose escalation trials (H0407g and H0452g) of single and weekly-repeated doses of Herceptin monotherapy were conducted in patients with advanced refractory HER2-positive metastatic breast cancer [Shak 1999]. In addition, two phase II trials of Herceptin monotherapy [Baselga et al. 1996] and Herceptin in combination with cisplatin [Pegram et al. 1998] were undertaken. As in the phase I trials, the patient population consisted of heavily pretreated HER2-positive metastatic breast cancer patients. These studies confirmed appropriate dosage, safety and potential efficacy of Herceptin as a single agent and in combination with concomitant chemotherapy in humans. Based on these data, progression to pivotal clinical trials was justified.

Two pivotal trials were conducted in large numbers of HER2-positive metastatic breast cancer patients: a phase II trial of second-/third-line Herceptin monotherapy (H0649g) [Cobleigh et al. 1999]; and a phase III first-line Herceptin combination trial (H0648g) [Mass et al. 2000; Norton et al. 1999; Slamon et al. 1998, 2001]. Details of these trials are described elsewhere [Baselga 2001; Mass et al. 2000; Shak 1999; Slamon et al. 2001]. In brief, Herceptin was administered as a 4-mg/kg initial dose followed by a 2-mg/kg i.v. weekly maintenance dose. In the combination trial, patients were randomized to receive Herceptin plus anthracycline/cyclophosphamide (AC) versus AC alone or, if they had previously received adjuvant anthracyclines, Herceptin plus paclitaxel versus paclitaxel alone.

In both trials Herceptin was well tolerated. Adverse events were generally mild to moderate and mainly associated with the first infusion. Cardiotoxicity was the most significant serious adverse event, particularly in patients receiving concomitant anthracyclines. However, in most cases this serious adverse event was manageable with standard medical treatment.

An independent Response Evaluation Committee (REC) determined tumor responses in the intent-to-treat-population (n = 222) of the pivotal phase II trial. They found an overall response rate of 15%, duration of response of 9.1 months and a median survival of 13 months. The median time to treatment failure (TTF) was 11 months which compared favorably with that for the prior regimen of chemotherapy (5.4 months).

Results for the pivotal combination trial were assessed at median 35 months follow-up. The primary endpoint of the trial, time to disease progression (TTP), was significantly improved in the Herceptin plus chemotherapy group compared with the chemotherapy alone group (7.4 versus 4.6 months). In addition, response rates, median duration of response and TTF were all significantly higher in the Herceptin plus chemotherapy group compared with the chemotherapy alone group. Of particular note, median survival duration was significantly increased from 20 months to 25 months by the addition of Herceptin to chemotherapy.

Following on from the pivotal trials, a phase II trial of Herceptin monotherapy was initiated in HER2-positive breast cancer patients who had not received prior chemotherapy for metastatic disease.

First-line Herceptin Monotherapy Trial

Study Design

In total, 114 women with HER2-positive metastatic breast cancer were enrolled into the multicenter, randomized trial [Vogel et al. 2000]. Enrollment closed May 1998. Patients were randomly assigned to one of two Herceptin dosing schedules, either: standard dose of 4 mg/kg initial dose followed by 2 mg/kg i.v. weekly, or high dose of 8 mg/kg initial dose followed by 4 mg/kg i.v. weekly. Treatment continued until disease progression.

Study Rationale

The primary objectives of the trial were to evaluate overall response rates and safety of first-line Herceptin monotherapy in each dose group. Tumor responses were assessed by the investigators at weeks 8, 16, 24 and every 12 weeks thereafter. Unlike the pivotal phase II monotherapy trial, an independent Response Evaluation Committee (REC) was not additionally employed to assess tumor responses in this study. An independent Cardiac Review Evaluation Committee (CREC) evaluated potential cases of cardiac dysfunction and safety was assessed by the investigators on a weekly basis. Secondary endpoints of the trial were duration of response, TTP, duration of survival and quality of life (QoL).

Patient Demographics/Eligibility

The patients enrolled in this trial were women with progressive breast cancer who did not wish to receive cytotoxic chemotherapy for metastatic disease. Eligible patients had not received prior chemotherapy for stage IV disease. In addition, patients had to have measurable disease; patients with bone-only lesions were excluded. HER2 status was determined by immunohistochemistry (IHC) and only IHC 2+ or 3+ patients were included in the study. The study protocol stipulated that Karnofsky Performance Status (KPS) had to be ≥70%, although 75% of patients enrolled in the study had a KPS of >80%.

At a median follow-up of 19 months (range 1.2 to 45.9 months) 3 of 114 patients were inevaluable: 1 patient received only one dose of Herceptin; 1 patient received four doses of Herceptin but did not have a post-baseline evaluation; the third patient did not have evidence of metastatic disease. Of the 111 evaluable patients, 58 were randomized to the standard Herceptin dose group and 53 were randomized to the high Herceptin dose group. Generally, patient demographics were comparable between the two dose groups. The mean age of patients was 54 years (range 28 to 86 years). Approximately half (52%) of the patients were estrogen receptor (ER) negative and approximately three-quarters (76%) were IHC 3+ HER2 overexpressors. Of those patients for whom fluorescence in situ hybridization (FISH) results were available (n = 62), more than half (41 of 62 patients) were FISH positive for HER2 overexpression. Twenty-eight percent of patients had a disease-free interval of ≤12 months. Approximately one third (31%) of patients had ≥ 3 metastatic sites and 67% had metastases of the liver and lung; 10% of patients demonstrated superficial metastases only. Patients had received prior adjuvant therapy for breast cancer including: chemotherapy (68%), anthracyclines (51%), and transplants (13%). In addition, 46% had received prior radiotherapy and 37% hormonal therapy.

Efficacy

The overall response rate (ORR) for first-line Herceptin monotherapy (ITT analysis) was 26% (95% CI: 18 to 34%) including 7 complete responses (CR) and 23 partial responses (PR). A further 13 patients had stable disease (SD) lasting >6 months for an overall clinical benefit (CR plus PR plus SD) of 38% (95% CI: 29 to 47%). Response rates were similar in the two dose groups for evaluable patients (table 1). The overall response rate was 24% (95% CI: 13 to 35%) [3 CR and 11 PR] in the standard-dose group compared with 28% (95% CI: 16 to 40% [4 CR and 11 PR] in the high-dose group.

Subset analysis demonstrated that, as expected, the response rate was quantitatively higher in patients with superficial metastases only. However, responses were also demonstrated in patients with liver or lung metastases. These response rates were particularly impressive if the definition of response included those patients with SD >6 months. Approximately one-third of patients demonstrated a response regardless of whether prior adjuvant therapy consisted of doxorubicin chemotherapy or stem cell transplantation.

Of particular note, the ORR was higher in the IHC 3+ subgroup (35%) compared with the overall (IHC 2+ and 3+) group (table 2). Interestingly, all responses (CR plus PR) were demonstrated in the IHC 3+ group, although 7% of IHC 2+ patients achieved SD >6 months.

Recent data have demonstrated that IHC and FISH are 82% concordant overall [Mass et al. 2000]. While IHC 3+ and FISH are highly concordant (89%), only 24% of

Table 1. Response rate by dose in evaluable patients following first-line single-agent Herceptin

	Number of patients	
	2 mg/kg	4 mg/kg
Treated	58	53
Complete response (CR)	3	4
Partial response (PR)	11	11
CR + PR	14 (24%) (95% CI 13–35%)	15 (28%) (95% CI 16–40%)

Table 2. Response according to HER2 status following first-line single-agent Herceptin

	Number of patients*	
	FISH+	FISH–
Response	17/41 (41%)	1/21 (5%)
Response rates, % (95% CI)		
FISH+	41 (26–56%)	
IHC 3+	35 (24–44%)	
IHC 2+ or 3+	26 (18–34%)	

* FISH results were available for 62 of 114 patients.

Table 3. Adverse events by dose group following first-line single-agent Herceptin

	Incidence, % patients			
	2 mg/kg (n = 59)		4 mg/kg (n = 55)	
	all	severe	all	severe
Pain	59	8	58	9
Asthenia	53	7	58	7
Fever	36	2	45	0
Nausea	37	3	47	2
Diarrhea	36	2	24	5
Headache	29	3	38	2
Chills	22	0	40	2
Rash	20	0	38	0
Rhinitis (epistaxis)	20 (12)	0	18 (7)	0
Dyspnea	15	0	25	2

IHC 2+ tumors are FISH positive. Analysis of response rates in patients for whom FISH results were available (n = 62) in the first-line Herceptin monotherapy trial, demonstrated that all but one objective response occurred in FISH-positive patients. The exception was a patient who was 3+ by IHC (a single-copy overexpressor). Response rates were 41% in FISH-positive patients compared with 5% in FISH-negative patients (table 2). Although not statistically significant, these data suggest a greater clinical benefit for FISH-positive compared with IHC 2+ and 3+ patients combined. When patients achieving stable disease for ≥6 months are added to the responders, the clinical benefit rate in IHC 3+ patients was 47%.

At a median follow-up of 9 months, 21 patients had not reached disease progression at the time of analysis. In responding patients (CR plus PR) median TTP was 18.8 months. For those patients not achieving a clinical benefit, median TTP was 1.8 months. Median duration of survival was 24.4 months (range 1.2 to 45.8+ months).

Safety

Herceptin was generally well tolerated as first-line monotherapy. As found in the pivotal Herceptin trials, most adverse events were mild to moderate and typically associated with the first infusion, rarely occurring with subsequent infusions. The most common adverse events were pain, asthenia, fever and chills. Overall, the incidence of adverse events was similar between the two Herceptin dose groups. However, acute infusion-related events such as fever and chills, as well as rash and dyspnea tended to occur more frequently with the higher dose schedule (table 3). Statistical analysis is required to determine whether this difference is significant. Adverse events typically associated with cytotoxic agents were rare in this study: alopecia 7%, leukopenia 4%, thrombocytopenia 1%, anemia 3%, and stomatitis 2%. In addition, assessment using the EORTC QLQ-C30 questionnaire demonstrated that most patients had either clinically meaningful improvements or no change in health-related QoL after beginning Herceptin monotherapy [Osoba et al. 2000].

Reports of serious cardiac events in the pivotal phase II and III Herceptin trials [Cobleigh et al. 1999; Cook-Bruns 2001; Ewer et al. 1999] prompted a retrospective analysis of cardiac events in this trial by an independent, blinded CREC. Cardiac dysfunction was defined by the CREC as symptomatic heart failure or an asymptomatic decrease (<10%) in left ventricular ejection fraction (LVEF). According to these criteria, three patients (2.6%) were identified as experiencing cardiac dysfunction, although one of these cases was not related to Herceptin therapy. In the remaining two patients, Herceptin therapy was discontinued after approximately 1 year.

There were 65 deaths, 34 in the standard Herceptin dose group and 31 in the high Herceptin dose group. None of these deaths occurred during the study and all deaths were due to progressive metastatic breast cancer.

Cross-Trial Comparisons

Although it is normally not possible to compare different trials with statistical accuracy, the first-line Herceptin monotherapy trial and the pivotal first-line Herceptin combination trial (H0648g) had the same investigators, similar patient populations and were run in parallel. Therefore, it is possible to compare these two trials in a cross-trial analysis with a view to identifying general trends between them.

In terms of patient demographics such as mean age, KPS, number of metastatic sites and HER2 positivity, there was virtually no difference between patients enrolled into each trial. However, differences were seen between the two trials in terms of the prior adjuvant chemotherapy patients had received. By nature of the trial design, the majority of patients in the Herceptin plus paclitaxel arm of the pivotal combination trial had received prior adjuvant doxorubicin (97%), while only 1% of patients had received prior doxorubicin in the Herceptin plus AC arm of this trial. In contrast, 51% of patients in the first-line monotherapy trial had received prior doxorubicin.

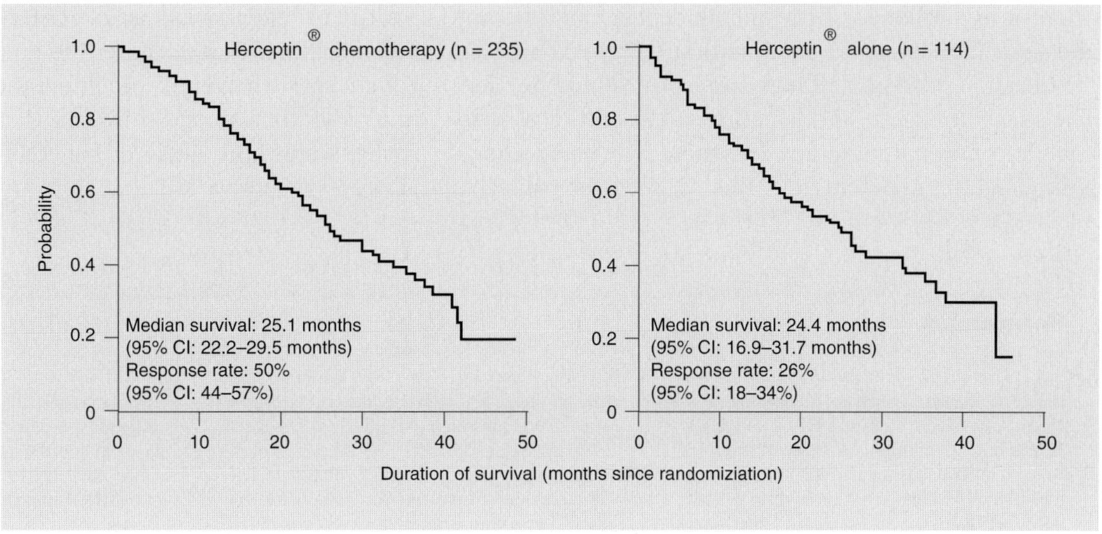

Fig. 1. Duration of survival following Herceptin plus chemotherapy (H0648g) or first-line Herceptin monotherapy.

These differences aside, comparison of Kaplan-Meier estimates of survival demonstrates similar survival duration between the two trials. Median survival for first-line Herceptin monotherapy was 24.4 months compared with 25.1 months for Herceptin plus chemotherapy (fig. 1). Similar survival rates were also seen between first-line Herceptin monotherapy and Herceptin plus paclitaxel (24.4 versus 22.1 months, respectively) and Herceptin plus AC (24.4 versus 26.8 months, respectively). However, response rates for Herceptin monotherapy were approximately half those of the combination therapy.

Analysis of outcomes in the two trials based on FISH data shows that not only is survival rate comparable between the two trials for FISH-positive patients (22.9 versus 26.8 months for first-line Herceptin monotherapy versus Herceptin plus chemotherapy, respectively) but that response rates are also similar (41% for first-line Herceptin monotherapy versus 54% for Herceptin plus chemotherapy).

Conclusions

The results from the first-line monotherapy trial demonstrate that Herceptin is active as a single agent in HER2-positive breast cancer patients who have not received prior therapy for metastatic disease. Importantly, efficacy was not improved by increasing the dose of Herceptin. A greater clinical benefit was observed in IHC 3+ patients than in the overall population, a trend which has also been demonstrated in the pivotal Herceptin trials [Baselga 2000; Mass et al. 2000].

Herceptin was well tolerated as first-line monotherapy and demonstrated a favorable safety profile. The incidence of cardiotoxicity also appeared to be lower in this study than in previously reported Herceptin trials, where the incidence of prior anthracycline exposure was greater. Moreover, based on the similar safety profile seen between the two dose groups in this study, it seems unlikely that Herceptin-associated adverse events are dose related, with a few possible exceptions. Therefore, since both efficacy and safety were similar between the two dose groups, the standard Herceptin dose (4 mg/kg initial dose followed by 2 mg/kg i.v. weekly maintenance dose), which was also the dose used in the pivotal trials, would be the preferred dosing schedule.

The results from this study indicate that FISH may offer a more accurate means of patient selection than IHC. Similar conclusions have also been drawn from the analysis of outcomes based on FISH positivity in the pivotal Herceptin trials [Baselga 2000; Mass et al. 2000]. It is likely that FISH allows the selection of all HER2 high overexpressors (including 24% of IHC 2+ patients) who are most likely to benefit from Herceptin therapy.

It is not possible to directly compare individual trials and deduce statistically significant conclusions about similarities. However, a comparison between the first-line Herceptin monotherapy and first-line Herceptin combination therapy trials does suggest that, although response rates are higher in the combination trial, overall survival duration is similar for first-line Herceptin monotherapy and first-line Herceptin combination therapy. This begs the question of when and how Herceptin should be used. The survival benefit and superior safety profile of first-line Herceptin monotherapy compared with chemotherapy highlights the potential of this regimen for palliative treatment of women with HER2-positive metastatic breast cancer. Furthermore, the greater level of clinical benefit seen when Herceptin monotherapy is used as first-line rather than second/third-line treatment indicates that patients are more likely to benefit from up-front use of Herceptin therapy.

References

Baselga J, Tripathy D, Mendelsohn J, Baughman S, Benz CC, Dantis L, Sklarin NT, Seidman AD, Hudis CA, Moore J, Rosen RP, Twaddell T, Henderson IC, Norton L: Phase II study of weekly intravenous recombinant humanized anti-p185^{HER2} monoclonal antibody in patients with HER2/*neu*-overexpressing metastatic breast cancer. J Clin Oncol 1996;14:737–744.

Baselga J, Norton L, Abanell J, Kim Y-M, Mendelsohn J: Recombinant humanized anti-HER2 antibody (Herceptin™) enhances the antitumor activity of paclitaxel and doxorubicin against HER2/*neu* overexpressing human breast cancer xenografts. Cancer Res 1998;58: 2825–2831.

Baselga J: Herceptin® alone or in combination with chemotherapy in the treatment of HER2-positive metastatic breast cancer: pivotal trials. Oncology 2001;61(suppl 2):14–21.

Benz CC, Scott, GK, Sarup JC, Johnson RM, Tripathy D, Coronado E, Shepard HM, Osborne CK: Estrogen-dependent, tamoxifen-resistant tumorigenic growth of MCF-7 cells transfected with HER2/*neu*. Breast Cancer Res Treat 1992;24:85–95.

Carter P, Presta L Gorman CM, Ridgway JB, Henner D, Wong WL, Rowland AM, Kotts C, Carver ME, Shepard HM: Humanization of an anti-p185HER2 antibody for human cancer therapy. Proc Natl Acad Sci USA 1992;89: 4285–4289.

Cobleigh MA, Vogel CL, Triapthy D, Robert NJ, Scholl, Fehrenbacher L, Wolter JM, Paton V, Shak S, Lieberman, Slamon DJ: Multinational study of the efficacy and safety of humanized anti-HER2 monoclonal antibody in women who have HER2-overexpressing metastatic breast cancer that has progressed after chemotherapy for metastatic disease. J Clin Oncol 1999;17:2639–2648.

Cook-Bruns N: Retrospective analysis of the safety of Herceptin® immunotherapy in metastatic breast cancer. Oncology 2001;61(suppl 2):58–66.

Di Fiore PP, Pierce JH, Fleming TP, Hazan R, Ullrich A, King CR, Schlessinger J, Aaronson SA: Overexpression of the human EGF receptor confers an EGF-dependent transformed phenotype to NIH 3T3 cells. Cell 1987a;51:1063–1070.

Di Fiore PP, Pierce JH, Kraus MH, Seatto O, King CR, Aaronson SA: *erb*B-2 is a potent oncogene when overexpressed in NIH/3T3 cells. Science 1987b;237:178–182.

Ewer MS, Gibbs HR, Swafford J, Benjamin RS: Cardiotoxicity in patients receiving Trastuzumab (Herceptin): primary toxicity, synergistic or sequential stress, or surveilance artifact? Semin Oncol 1999;26(suppl 12):96–101.

Hortobagyi GN: Treatment of breast cancer. N Engl J Med 1998;339:974–984.

Hudziak RM, Schlessinger J, Ullrich A. Increased expression of the putative growth factor receptor p185^{HER2} causes transformation and tumorigenesis of NIH 3T3 cells. Proc Natl Acad Sci USA 1987;84:7159–7163.

Landis SH, Murray T, Bolden S, Wingo PA: Cancer statistics, 1999. CA Cancer J Clin 1999;49:8–31.

Lewis GD, Fiagari I, Fendly B, Wong WL, Carter P, Gormon C, Shepard HM: Differential responses of the human tumor cell lines to anti-p185^{HER2} monoclonal antibodies. Cancer Immunol Immunother 1993;37:255–263.

Mass RD, Sanders C, Charlene K, Johnson L, Everett T, Anderson S: The concordance between the clinical trials assay (CTA) and fluorescence in situ hybridization (FISH) in the Herceptin pivotal trials. Proc Am Soc Clin Oncol 2000; 19:75A.

Norton L, Slamon D, Leyland-Jones B, Wolter J, Fleming T, Eiermann W, Baselga J, Mendelsohn J, Bajamonde A, Ash M, Shak S: Overall survival (OS) advantage to simultaneous chemotherapy (Crx) plus the humanized anti-HER2 monoclonal antibody Herceptin (H) in HER2-overexpressing (HER2+) metastatic breast cancer (MBC). Proc Am Soc Clin Oncol 1999;18:127A.

Osoba D, Burchmore, M, Ash, M, Tripathy D, Vogel C: Health related quality of life (HRQL) of patients with first-line, single-agent, Trastuzumab (Herceptin) for metastatic HER-2 overexpressing breast cancer. Proc Am Soc Clin Oncol 2000;19:436A.

Pegram MD, Pietras RJ, Slamon DJ: Monoclonal antibody to HER-2/neu gene product potentiates cytotoxicity of carboplatin and doxorubicin in human breast tumor cells. Proc Am Assoc Cancer Res 1992;33:442.

Pegram MD, Finn RS, Arzoo K, Beryt M, Pietras RJ, Slamon DJ: The effect of HER-2/neu overexpression on chemotherapeutic drug sensitivity in human breast and ovarian cancer cells. Oncogene 1997;15:537–547.

Pegram MD, Lipton, A, Hayes DF, Weber BL, Baselga JM, Tripathy D, Baly D, Baughman SA, Twaddell T, Glapsy JA, Slamon DJ: Phase II study of receptor-enhanced chemosensitivity using recombinant humanized anti-p18 5HER2/*neu* monoclonal antibody plus cisplatin in patients with HER2/*neu*-overexpressing metastatic breast cancer refractory to chemotherapy treatment. J Clin Oncol 1998;16:2659–2671.

Pegram M, Hsu S, Lewis G, Pietras R, Beryt M, Sliwkowski M, Coombs D, Baly D, Kabbinavar F, Slaomn D: Inhibitory effects of combinations of HER-2/*neu* antibody and chemotherapeutic agents used for treatment of human breast cancers. Oncogene 1999;18:2241–2251.

Shak S: Overview of the trastuzumab (Herceptin) anti-HER2 monoclonal antibody clinical program in HER2-overexpressing metastatic breast cancer. Semin Oncol 1999;26(suppl 12): 71–77.

Slamon D, et al. Leyland-Jones B, Shak S, Paton V, Bajamonde A, Fleming T, Eiermann W, Wolter J, Baselga J, Norton L: Addition of Herceptin™ (humanized anti-HER2 antibody) to first line chemotherapy for HER2 overexpressing metastatic breast cancer (HER2+/MBC) markedly increases anticancer activity: a randomized, multinational controlled phase III trial. Proc Am Soc Clin Oncol 1998;17:98A.

Slamon DJ, Leyland-Jones B, Shak S, Fuchs H, Paton V, Bajamonde A, Fleming T, Eiermann W, Wolter J, Pegram M, Baselga J, Norton L: Use of chemotherapy plus a monoclonal antibody against HER2 for metastatic breast cancer that overexpresses HER2. N Engl J Med 2001;344:783–792.

Vogel C, Cobleigh M, Tripathy D, Harris L, Fehrenbacher L, Slamon D, Ash M, Novotny W, Stewart S, Shak S: First-line, non-hormonal, treatment of woman with HER2 overexpressing metastatic breast cancer with Herceptin (Trastuzumab, humanized anti-HER2 antibody). Proc Am Soc Clin Oncol 2000;19:71A.

Oncology

Oncology 2001;61(suppl 2):43–49

Interaction between Herceptin® and Taxanes

Véronique Diéras P. Beuzeboc V. Laurence J.Y. Pierga P. Pouillart

Department of Medical Oncology, Institut Curie, Service de Medecine Oncologique, Paris, France

Key Words

Herceptin® · Taxanes · Paclitaxel · Docetaxel · HER2 · Metastatic breast cancer

Abstract

The taxanes and Herceptin® have been shown to possess significant clinical activity in metastatic breast cancer. Preclinical testing of taxane/Herceptin combinations demonstrated additive and synergistic interactions with paclitaxel and docetaxel, respectively. In a pivotal clinical trial, combination of paclitaxel (3-weekly) and Herceptin was associated with an increased response rate compared with paclitaxel monotherapy (41% vs. 17%; p = 0.001). The combination therapy also significantly improved time to disease progression (6.9 vs. 2.7 months; $p < 0.05$). In a phase II study of weekly paclitaxel plus Herceptin in patients with normal or increased tumor HER2 levels, a response was observed in 60% of patients and the regimen was well tolerated. Responses were more frequent in patients with HER2-overexpressing tumors (83% vs. 45%). Preliminary results from a phase II study of Herceptin plus docetaxel in patients with HER2-overexpressing tumors indicate significant activity, with a response observed in 7 (44%) of 16 evaluable patients. The preliminary results of a trial of weekly docetaxel and Herceptin demonstrate a response rate of 54% in 13 evaluable patients. Additional European trials of Herceptin/taxane combinations as first- and second-line and adjuvant therapy are ongoing. The results of the studies to date indicate that regimens combining Herceptin with 3-weekly and weekly taxane are effective and well tolerated.

Introduction

Herceptin® is a humanized monoclonal antibody (MAb) directed against the HER2 protein, which is overexpressed in a number of different human cancers [Salomon et al. 1995]. The results of small phase II trials established that Herceptin is a well-tolerated and clinically active treatment in women with HER2-overexpressing metastatic breast cancer [Baselga et al. 1996; Pegram et al. 1998]. A large phase II pivotal trial recently evaluated the use of Herceptin as a second/third-line agent for treatment of HER2-positive patients with metastatic breast cancer [Cobleigh et al. 1999]. In this trial, which included 222 women, patients received an initial i.v. dose of 4 mg/kg, followed by a 2 mg/kg maintenance dose at weekly intervals. The overall response rate was determined to be 15% with a median duration of response of 9.1 months. The encouraging results of this pivotal trial in part led to the approval of Herceptin by the United States Food and Drug Administration (US FDA) for treatment

KARGER

Fax +41 61 306 12 34
E-Mail karger@karger.ch
www.karger.com

0030–2414/01/0616–0043$17.50/0

Accessible online at:
www.karger.com/journals/ocl

V. Diéras, MD
Institut Curie, Service de Medecine Oncologique
F–75005 Paris (France)
Tel. +33 1 44 32 46 81, Fax +33 1 44 32 46 77
E-Mail veronique.dieras@curie.net

of relapsed, metastatic, HER2-overexpressing breast cancer in the USA [Brenner and Adams 1999].

The taxanes, paclitaxel and docetaxel, represent two of the most active chemotherapeutic agents for the treatment of patients with breast cancer [Harris et al. 1997]. These novel, diterpene chemotherapeutic agents act by inhibiting microtubule disassembly. Paclitaxel was the first diterpene agent to be developed for clinical use and has demonstrated activity in the treatment of a number of different human cancers [Rowinsky 1997]. Paclitaxel is active in the treatment of metastatic breast cancer as first-line therapy, where it is associated with response rates of 20 to 30% [Davidson 1996; Seidman et al. 1995a]. Paclitaxel therapy also plays an important role in the treatment of heavily pretreated patients [Abrams et al. 1995; Seidman et al. 1995a, b]. Of note, a response rate of approximately 23% was reported for anthracycline-resistant patients [Abrams et al. 1995]. Docetaxel has been demonstrated to possess high activity in the treatment of metastatic breast cancer. In a series of three phase II studies in first-line treatment of metastatic breast cancer, an overall response rate of 56% was seen in 117 patients [Fumoleau et al. 1996; Hudis et al. 1996; Trudeau et al. 1996]. In a similar number of second-line patients, the response rate was 49% [Ravdin et al. 1995; Ravdin 1996; ten Bokkel Huinink et al. 1994; Valero et al. 1995] and, of note, was 42% in the 105 patients defined as anthracycline-resistant [Guastalla et al. 1995; Ravdin et al. 1995; Ravdin 1996; Valero et al. 1995].

Combination chemotherapy is frequently used for the treatment of advanced breast cancer. Multidrug regimens have generally resulted in higher complete and overall response rates, with improvements in response duration. The rationale for combination therapies resides in the individual activities of the agents, the differing molecular targets for the mechanisms of action, and nonoverlapping toxicity profiles. Herceptin has been demonstrated to enhance the cytotoxic activity of cisplatin in vitro [Hancock et al. 1991; Pietras et al. 1994]. Furthermore, there has been one report indicating that HER2 overexpression predicts for sensitivity to taxane therapy [Baselga et al. 1997], indicating that tumors suitable for treatment with Herceptin may also be ideal targets for taxane therapy. Additional studies are, however, warranted to confirm this potential predictive value of HER2 with respect to taxane therapy.

The excellent clinical activities of the taxanes, paclitaxel and docetaxel, identify them as promising candidate agents for combination with Herceptin. Indeed, therapies comprising Herceptin/paclitaxel and Herceptin/docetaxel combinations are already generating promising data. This paper describes the major trials that are ongoing to evaluate Herceptin in combination with the taxanes in metastatic breast cancer, and provides a brief overview of the many smaller Herceptin plus taxane trials underway.

Combination of Paclitaxel and Herceptin

In vitro studies to define the interactions between clinically relevant concentrations of Herceptin and a range of cytotoxic drugs (using a multiple drug effect/combination index (CI) isobologram analysis) demonstrated an additive effect for the combination of Herceptin and paclitaxel [Pegram et al. 1999]. A preclinical study has also demonstrated a capacity for Herceptin to enhance the antitumor activity of paclitaxel against HER2-overexpressing tumors [Baselga et al. 1998]. In this study, the addition of Herceptin produced an additive and concentration-dependent effect on the cytotoxicity of paclitaxel in cultures of human carcinoma cell lines overexpressing HER2. The combination yielded a striking rate of tumor eradication in a nude mouse model, and thus provided further evidence that Herceptin can effectively enhance the tumoricidal effects of paclitaxel. Following a 5-week treatment period, 59% of mice who had received Herceptin and paclitaxel were tumor free, compared with 17.3% of mice treated with paclitaxel alone ($p = 0.004$). This effect was greater than that observed with doxorubicin, where combination with Herceptin yielded 33.3% tumor-free mice, compared with 13% treated with doxorubicin alone ($p = 0.09$). The increased effects were observed in the absence of additional animal toxicity. The mechanisms underlying the interaction between paclitaxel and Herceptin remain unelucidated and may be simply a summation of the individual activities of two anticancer agents that act at different targets.

In a recent pivotal, multicenter phase III trial of Herceptin in combination with chemotherapy (H0648g) as first-line treatment for HER2-positive metastatic breast cancer, a total of 469 patients were randomized to receive chemotherapy alone or chemotherapy plus Herceptin [Norton et al. 1999; Slamon et al. 2001]. Patients who had received no prior anthracyclines received anthracycline plus cyclophosphamide (AC) alone or in combination with Herceptin ($n = 281$). Patients previously given anthracyclines ($n = 188$) received paclitaxel alone or in combination with Herceptin. At a median follow-up of 35 months, the overall response rate and median time to progression (TTP) in the Herceptin group were 50% and 7.4

months, respectively. These results were superior to those observed in the group who received chemotherapy alone (response rate, 32%; median time to progression, 4.6 months; $p < 0.05$). Specifically with paclitaxel, the overall response rate with Herceptin was 41%, with a TTP of 6.9%, which was statistically greater than that observed with paclitaxel alone (response rate, 17%; TTP 2.7 months; $p < 0.05$). Addition of Herceptin to chemotherapy was associated with a significant increase in overall survival compared with chemotherapy alone (25 vs. 20 months; $p < 0.05$). The overall survival advantage for addition of Herceptin was maintained in the paclitaxel subgroup (22 vs. 18 months).

Table 1. Phase II study of Herceptin plus weekly paclitaxel – patient characteristics

Number of patients	95
Median age, years (range)	51 years (28–68)
Median Karnofsky performance status (range)	90% (70–100)
Median No. organ systems with metastases	2 (1–6)
Visceral dominant disease	87%
Prior chemotherapy	
Adjuvant	77%
Metastatic	31%
1 regimen	18%
≥2 regimens	13%
Prior anthracycline	65%
Prior taxane (>1 year)	13%
Prior high dose chemotherapy	2%

Weekly Paclitaxel and Herceptin

Paclitaxel is commonly administered using a 3-hour infusion at a dose of 135–250 mg/m^2 every three weeks. However, there is currently much interest in the administration of weekly cycles of paclitaxel. Weekly administration of moderate doses of paclitaxel is associated with higher cumulative doses with little effect on toxicity [Baselga et al. 1998; Norton et al. 1999; Pegram et al. 1999; Seidman 1998; Seidman et al. 2000]. Seidman and coworkers [Seidman 1998] conducted a study of paclitaxel (100 mg/m^2) administered weekly via 1-hour infusion to patients with previously treated metastatic breast cancer. This monotherapy produced a 53% response rate, including 10% complete responses. Of note, a response rate of 50% was observed in the subgroup of patients with anthracycline-resistant disease. These data, taken together with the observed survival advantage for patients receiving Herceptin/paclitaxel combination therapy, lent support to the development of a regimen combining Herceptin and weekly (dose-dense) paclitaxel.

Thus, a follow-up phase II study was conducted to evaluate the safety and therapeutic efficacy of dose-dense paclitaxel and Herceptin in HER2-positive and -negative patients with metastatic breast cancer [Seidman et al. 2000]. Herceptin was administered as an initial dose of 4 mg/kg over 90 min on week 1, followed by 2 mg/kg over 30 min on subsequent weeks. Paclitaxel was given at a dose of 90 mg/m^2 over 60 min weekly. A total of 95 patients with a median age of 51 years (range 28–68 years) and median Karnofsky Performance Status (KPS) of 90% (range 70–100) received treatment (table 1). The median number of organ systems affected by metastases was 2 (1–6) and visceral dominant disease was present in 87% of patients. Patients had received a maximum of three previous chemotherapy regimens; 77% had received prior adjuvant treatment and 31% chemotherapy for metastatic disease (18%, 1 regimen; 13%, 2 regimens) including: anthracyclines (65%), taxanes (13%), and high-dose therapy (2%). The HER2 status of tumors was determined by immunohistochemistry (IHC) using the DAKO HercepTest®, P-Ab1, TAB-250 or CB-11. In addition, HER2 gene amplification was assessed by fluorescence in situ hybridization (FISH) using the PathVysion™ kit from Vysis.

More than 2,600 infusions of Herceptin and paclitaxel were administered and the median number for each patient was 25 (1–85). The dose intensity of paclitaxel was good and the median paclitaxel delivered dose intensity was 82 mg/m^2/week (range 52–90). Importantly, the combination therapy was well tolerated, with a toxicity profile similar to that of paclitaxel alone. Neuropathy was the major dose-limiting adverse effect, with grade 3/4 neuropathy observed in 11% of patients. Although grade 3/4 neutropenia was observed in 14% of patients, there were, however, only 3 episodes of febrile neutropenia. Signs and symptoms of cardiac dysfunction had been noted in some patients on the Herceptin and paclitaxel arm of the pivotal phase III trial [Norton et al. 1999; Slamon et al. 1998]. For this reason, cardiac symptoms were monitored carefully in the weekly Herceptin plus paclitaxel trial. Congestive heart failure occurred in 2 patients, myocardial infarction in 2 patients, and serial ventriculography (MUGA) revealed a decline in left ventricular ejection fraction (LVEF) in 4 patients. However, even though some patients had a LVEF below 50% at baseline, cardiac function was preserved for up to a year in the majority of patients (fig. 1).

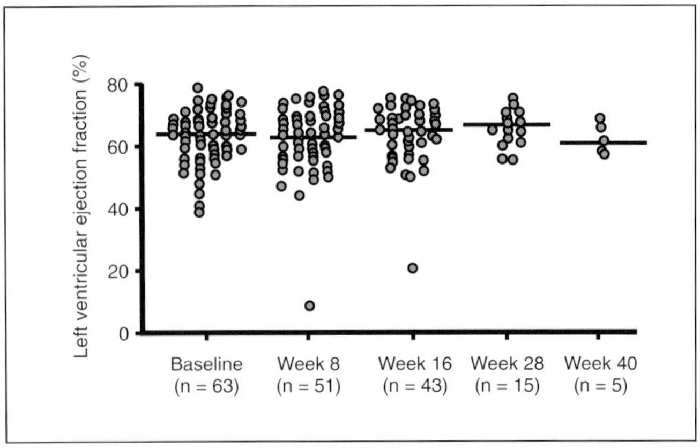

Fig. 1. Herceptin plus weekly paclitaxel – left ventricular function.

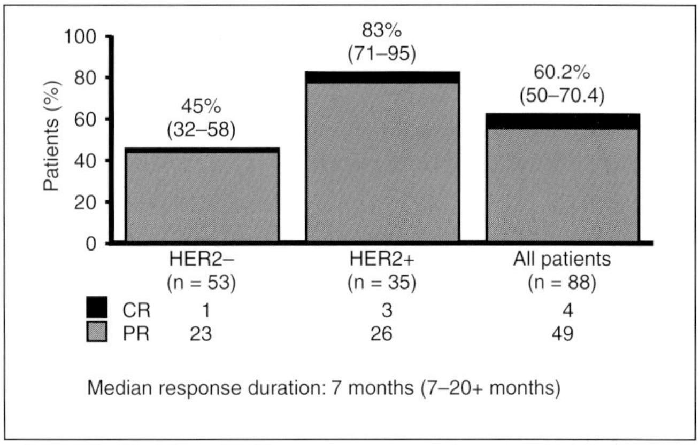

Fig. 2. Herceptin plus weekly paclitaxel – overall response rates according to HER2 expression levels.

A total of 88 patients were evaluable for efficacy and, of these, a response was observed in 53 (ORR 60%). The responses included 49 partial responses and 4 complete responses. Response rates were found to depend on HER2 status. Selection of HER2-positive patients using the MAb TAB250 was found to be the best approach to identifying patients who achieve a clinical response; responses were observed in 83% of TAB250-positive patients and 45% of TAB250-negative patients ($p = 0.001$) (fig. 2). A significant association between HER2 status and response to treatment was also demonstrated for MAb CB11 ($p = 0.006$). The roles of the DAKO HercepTest and P-Ab1 in the prediction of response to therapy were less clear because no statistically significant associations were demonstrated. HER2 gene amplification by FISH, however, was shown to be associated with response to treatment ($p = 0.01$). Of the 40 FISH-positive patients (45%), a response was observed in 30 (75%). Responses were also noted in 23 of 48 (48%) patients with no evidence of HER2 amplification. Overall, these data demonstrate that weekly Herceptin plus paclitaxel has significant clinical benefit and a favorable safety profile in HER2-positive patients.

A further study of weekly Herceptin plus paclitaxel in 19 patients with metastatic breast cancer and HER2-overexpressing tumors attending a private practice setting has produced promising results for this regimen [Yeung et al. 2000]. Patients received an initial dose of 4 mg/kg Herceptin followed by 2 mg/kg weekly in combination with 80 mg/m^2/week paclitaxel. Prior chemotherapy regimens had been administered to 95% of patients (1 regimen, 42%, 2 regimens, 26% and 3+ regimens 27%). A total of 7 (37%) patients had received prior taxane therapy. Objective responses were observed in 5 (27%) patients and included 3 complete responses. The median TTP was 23 weeks. Furthermore, the regimen was well tolerated and proved suitable for private practice.

The encouraging results from both trials have led to the integration of Herceptin into the phase III Cancer and Leukemia Group B (CALGB) study comparing dose-dense and conventional paclitaxel with or without Herceptin in patients (HER2-positive and HER2-negative) with inoperable, recurrent or metastatic breast cancer. A total of 580 patients will be accrued for this study within 3 years.

Furthermore, different dose schedules for Herceptin are currently being evaluated and a phase I/II trial to determine the safety and pharmacokinetics of Herceptin plus paclitaxel in a 3-weekly combination in women with metastatic breast cancer is being conducted [Leyland-Jones et al. 2000a, b].

Herceptin plus Docetaxel

Preclinical studies have demonstrated a synergistic interaction between docetaxel and Herceptin. Clinical evaluation of concomitant Herceptin plus docetaxel was therefore a logical development [Hortobagyi 1999]. A small phase II study to investigate the combination of Herceptin (4 mg/kg initial dose followed by 2 mg/kg until disease progression) plus docetaxel (75 mg/m^2, 3-weekly for 6 cycles) as first- or second-line therapy in HER2-overexpressing metastatic breast cancer is currently ongoing. All patients' tumor specimens were evaluated for HER2 expression levels using the HercepTest IHC assay, and those assessed as 2+ or 3+ are eligible for inclusion in the study. Preliminary results indicate significant activity, and 7 responses have been noted (1 complete response and 6 partial responses) in the 16 evaluable patients [Kuzur et al. 2000]. Six of the seven major responses were observed in the HER2 3+ subgroup, yielding response rates for the HER2 3+ and 2+ subgroups of 55% and 20%, respectively. To date, median time to progression exceeds 6 months. This combination regimen has been well tolerated, with no reports of serious toxicity and only one report of febrile neutropenia. Furthermore, no clinically significant cardiotoxicity has been observed.

A schedule including weekly administration of Herceptin and docetaxel is currently being investigated in HER2-positive patients with advanced breast cancer. Preliminary results from a pilot phase II study to investigate the safety and efficacy of weekly docetaxel (35 mg/m^2, 6 of 8 weeks) and weekly Herceptin (4 mg/kg initial dose followed by 2 mg/kg) as first- or second-line therapy have demonstrated significant activity. Of 13 evaluable patients, responses have been noted in 7 (1 complete response and 6 partial responses), yielding an overall response rate of 54% [Nicholson et al. 2000]. As is the case with patients receiving Herceptin plus paclitaxel, Herceptin plus docetaxel is proving to be well tolerated with a toxicity profile similar to that of docetaxel alone, and appears to be an active therapeutic option.

Table 2. Additional taxane/Herceptin trials currently ongoing in Europe

Country	Trial	Patients
Europe-wide	Docetaxel ± Herceptin	156
Germany	Herceptin + docetaxel (weekly or 3-weekly)	100
Italy	Herceptin + epirubicin + docetaxel	60
Italy	Paclitaxel ± Herceptin	176

Table 3. Adjuvant trials of Herceptin plus taxanes

Collaborative group	Trial design
NSABP	AC→P vs. AC→P + H
Intergroup	AC→P vs. AC→P + H vs. AC→P→H
BCIRG	AC + docetaxel vs. AC + D + H vs. platinum + D + H

Other Ongoing Trials

Additional European trials of Herceptin in combination with taxanes are ongoing in patients with metastatic breast cancer (table 2), and include a phase III, multicenter registration trial to compare docetaxel monotherapy with docetaxel and Herceptin combination therapy in 156 patients with HER2-overexpressing tumors. Other trials will compare paclitaxel monotherapy with paclitaxel and Herceptin combination therapy, and weekly and 3-weekly paclitaxel in combination with Herceptin. In addition, an Italian trial will evaluate a combination of Herceptin, epirubicin and docetaxel.

A number of trials to evaluate the adjuvant role of Herceptin and taxane combination therapy have also commenced recruitment (table 3). The National Adjuvant Surgical Breast and Bowel Project (NSABP) trial will compare paclitaxel with a paclitaxel/Herceptin combination following prior anthracycline treatment. The Intergroup trial will address the same issue and will incorporate a third study arm with sequential anthracycline, paclitaxel and Herceptin therapies. A Breast Cancer International Research Group (BCIRG) trial will compare the following three regimens: anthracycline plus docetaxel; anthracycline plus docetaxel plus Herceptin; and platinum-based therapy in combination with docetaxel and Herceptin.

Conclusions

Combination chemotherapy is often employed in the treatment of metastatic breast cancer patients. Several clinical trials are currently exploring the therapeutic potential of therapies that combine the novel biological agent, Herceptin, with other anticancer agents with recognized therapeutic value. Paclitaxel and docetaxel are obvious candidates to evaluate in combination, and to date the major studies of combination therapy have centered on the efficacy of Herceptin in combination with various dose schedules of taxanes [Kuzur et al. 2000; Nicholson et al. 2000; Norton et al. 1999; Seidman et al. 2000]. The rationale for assessing Herceptin/taxane therapies is based on preclinical data indicating additive and synergistic antitumor efficacy of Herceptin plus paclitaxel and docetaxel, respectively [Baselga et al. 1998; Pegram et al.

1999], and the pivotal phase III clinical trial data demonstrating the significant therapeutic efficacy of first-line Herceptin plus paclitaxel in HER2-positive metastatic breast cancer [Norton et al. 1999; Slamon et al. 2001].

So far, studies assessing concomitant Herceptin plus taxane therapy provide additional support for the benefits observed in the pivotal phase III trial; addition of Herceptin to 1-hour paclitaxel as a weekly regimen has been shown to be an effective and well-tolerated regimen in metastatic breast cancer patients [Seidman et al. 2000]. In particular, HER2-positive patients showed an 83% response rate. The role of combined weekly Herceptin/paclitaxel therapy in HER2-negative patients, who obtained a 45% response rate, remains to be elucidated. A 27% response rate to weekly Herceptin plus 1-hour paclitaxel has been reported [Yeung et al. 2000]. A trial of 3-weekly Herceptin plus paclitaxel is also ongoing, the preliminary results from which appear promising [Leyland-Jones et al. 2000ab]. The reports from trials of weekly Herceptin plus docetaxel (weekly or 3-weekly) indicate that this combination is also active in metastatic breast cancer [Kuzur et al. 2000; Nicholson et al. 2000]. Importantly, the combined therapies containing either taxane have favorable safety profiles similar to those of the individual taxanes. Emerging data suggest that taxane/Herceptin combinations may find a role in adjuvant therapy for metastatic breast cancer [for a review, see Leyland-Jones and Smith 2001]. As more data emerge, it will be possible to further define the clinical role of Herceptin/taxane regimens.

References

Abrams JS, Vena DA, Baltz J, Montello M, Christian M, Onetto N, Desmond-Hellmann S, Canetta R, Friedman MA, et al: Paclitaxel activity in heavily pretreated breast cancer: A National Cancer Institute Treatment Referral Center Trial. J Clin Oncol 1995;13:2056–2065.

Baselga J, Norton L, Albanell J, Kim YM, Mendelsohn J: Recombinant humanized anti-HER2 antibody (Herceptin™) enhances the antitumor activity of paclitaxel and doxorubicin against HER2/neu overexpressing human breast cancer xenografts. Cancer Res 1998;58: 2825–2831.

Baselga J, Seidman AD, Rosen PP, Norton L: HER2 overexpression and paclitaxel sensitivity in breast cancer: therapeutic implications. Oncology (Huntingt) 1997;11(suppl 2):43–48.

Baselga J, Tripathy D, Mendelsohn J, Baughman S, Benz CC, Dantis L, Sklarin NT, Seidman AD, Hudis CA, Moore J, Rosen PP, Twaddell T, Henderson IC, Norton L: Phase II study of weekly intravenous recombinant humanized anti-p185HER2 monoclonal antibody in patients with HER2/neu-overexpressing metastatic breast cancer. J Clin Oncol 1996;14:737–744.

Brenner TL, Adams VR: First MAb approved for the treatment of metastatic breast cancer. J Am Pharm Assoc 1999;39:236–238.

Cobleigh MA, Vogel CL, Tripathy D, Robert NJ, Scholl S, Fehrenbacher L, Wolter JM, Paton V, Shak S, Lieberman G, Slamon DJ: Multinational study of the efficacy and safety of humanized anti-HER2 monoclonal antibody in women who have HER2-overexpressing metastatic breast cancer that has progressed after chemotherapy for metastatic disease. J Clin Oncol 1999;17:2639–2648.

Davidson NG: Single-agent paclitaxel as first-line treatment of metastatic breast cancer: the British experience. Semin Oncol 1996;23(suppl 11):6–10.

Fumoleau P, Chevallier B, Kerbrat P, Krakowski Y, Misset JL, Maugard-Louboutin C, Dieras V, Azli N, Bougon N, Riva A, Roche H: A multicentre phase II study of the efficacy and safety of docetaxel as first-line treatment of advanced breast cancer: report of the Clinical Screening Group of the EORTC. Ann Oncol 1996;7:165–171.

Guastalla JP, Bonnetterre J, Fumoleau P, Piccart M, Tubiana M, Chevallier B, Nieamann C, Alakl M, Nichol A, Riva A, Marty M: A phase II trial of docetaxel in patients with anthracycline-resistant metastatic breast cancer. Eur J Cancer 1995;31(suppl 5):S75–S77.

Hancock MC, Langton BC, Chan T, Toy P, Monahan JJ, Mischak RP, Shawver LK: A monoclonal antibody against the c-erbB-2 protein enhances the cytotoxicity of cis-diamminedichloroplatinum against human breast and ovarian tumor cell lines. Cancer Res 1991;51: 4575–4580.

Harris JR, Morrow M, Norton L: Malignant tumors of the breast; in DeVita VT, Hellman S and Rosenberg SA (eds): Cancer, Principles and Practice of Oncology, ed 5. Philadelphia, Lippincott-Raven, 1997, pp 1557–1616.

Hortobagyi GN: Recent progress in the clinical development of docetaxel. Semin Oncol 1999; 26(suppl 9):32–36.

Hudis CA, Seidman AD, Crown JP, Balmaceda C, Freilich R, Gilewski TA, Hakes TB, Currie V, Lebwohl DE, Baselga J, Raptis G, Gollub M, Robles M, Bruno R, Norton L: Phase II and pharmacologic study of docetaxel as initial chemotherapy for metastatic breast cancer. J Clin Oncol 1996;14:58–65.

Kuzur ME, Albain KS, Huntington MO, Jones SF, Hainsworth JD, Greco FA, Erland JB, Vogel CL, Burris HA: A phase II trial of docetaxel and Herceptin in metastatic breast cancer patients overexpressing HER-2. Proc Am Soc Clin Oncol 2000;19:131A.

Leyland-Jones B, Arnold A, Gelmon K, Verma S, Rakhit A, Howell J. A pharmacokinetic (PK) study of Herceptin® administered with paclitaxel i.v. every 3 weeks. Eur J Cancer 2000a; S35:abstract 41.

Leyland-Jones B, Hemmings F, Arnold A, Gelmon K, Verma S, Ayoub J-P. Pharmacokinetics of Herceptin® administered with paclitaxel every three weeks. Cancer Res Treat 2000b;124:abstract 534.

Leyland-Jones B, Smith I: Role of Herceptin® in primary breast cancer: Views from North America and Europe. Oncology 2001;61(suppl 2):83–91.

Nicholson BP, Thor AD, Goldstein LJ, Merkel DE, Gradishar WJ, Sledge GW: Weekly docetaxel (D) and Rhumabher2 (H) combination therapy as first- or second-line treatment for metastatic breast cancer (MBC). Proc Am Soc Clin Oncol 2000;19:139A.

Norton L, Slamon D, Leyland-Jones B, Wolter J, Fleming T, Eirmann W, Baselga J, Mendelsohn J, Bajamonde A, Ash M, Shak S: Overall survival (OS) advantage to simultaneous chemotherapy (CRx) plus humanized anti-HER2 monoclonal antibody herceptin (H) in HER2-overexpressing (HER2+) metastatic breast cancer (MBC). Proc Am Soc Clin Oncol 1999;18: 127A.

Pegram M, Hsu S, Lewis G, Pietras R, Beryt M, Sliwkowski M, Coombs D, Baly D, Kabbinavar F, Slamon D: Inhibitory effects of combinations of HER-2/neu antibody and chemotherapeutic agents used for treatment of human breast cancers. Oncogene 1999;18:2241–2251.

Pegram MD, Lipton A, Hayes DF, Weber BL, Baselga JM, Tripathy D, Baly D, Baughman SA, Twaddell T, Glaspy JA, Slamon DJ: Phase II study of receptor-enhanced chemosensitivity using recombinant humanized anti-p185HER2/neu monoclonal antibody plus cisplatin in patients with HER2/neu-overexpressing metastatic breast cancer refractory to chemotherapy treatment. J Clin Oncol 1998;16:2659–2671.
Pietras RJ, Fendly BM, Chazin VR, Pegram MD, Howell SB, Slamon DJ: Antibody to HER-2/neu receptor blocks DNA repair after cisplatin in human breast and ovarian cancer cells. Oncogene 1994;9:1829–1838.
Ravdin PM: Treatment of patients resistant to anthracycline therapy. Anticancer Drugs 1996;7(suppl 2):13–16.
Ravdin PM, Burris HA 3rd, Cook G, Eisenberg P, Kane M, Bierman WA, Mortimer J, Genevois E, Bellet RE: Phase II trial of docetaxel in advanced anthracycline-resistant or anthracenedione-resistant breast cancer. J Clin Oncol 1995;13:2879–2885.
Rowinsky EK: Paclitaxel pharmacology and other tumor types. Semin Oncol 1997;24(suppl 19):1–12.
Salomon DS, Brandt R, Ciardiello F, Normanno N: Epidermal growth factor-related peptides and their receptors in human malignancies. Crit Rev Oncol Hematol 1995;19:1183–1232.
Seidman AD, Fornier M, Esteva F, Tan L, Kaptain S, Bach A, Arroyo CD, Currie V, Gilewski T, Theodoulou M, Moynahan ME, Moasser M, D'Andrea G, Sklarin N, Dickler M, Chin J, Denton C, Bacotti D, Willey J, Frye D, Hortobagyi G, Norton L, Hudis C: Final report: weekly (W) Herceptin (H) and Taxol (T) for metastatic breast cancer (MBC): analysis of efficacy by HER2 immunophenotype [immunohistochemistry (IHC)] and gene amplification [fluorescence in-situ hybridization (FISH)]. Proc Am Soc Clin Oncol 2000;19:83A.
Seidman AD, Tiersten A, Hudis C, Gollub M, Barrett S, Yao TJ, Lepore J, Gilewski T, Currie V, Crown J, et al: Phase II trial of paclitaxel by 3-hour infusion as initial and salvage chemotherapy for metastatic breast cancer. J Clin Oncol 1995a;13:2575–2581.
Seidman AD, Reichman BS, Crown JP, Yao TJ, Currie V, Hakes TB, Hudis CA, Gilewski TA, Baselga J, Forsythe P, et al: Paclitaxel as second and subsequent therapy for metastatic breast cancer: activity independent of prior anthracycline response. J Clin Oncol 1995b;13:11152–11159.
Seidman AD: One hour paclitaxel via weekly infusion: dose-density with enhanced therapeutic index. Oncology 1998;12(suppl 1):19–22.
Slamon D, Leyland-Jones B, Shak S, Paton V, Bajamonde A, Fleming T, Eiermann W, Wolter J, Baselga J, Norton L: Use of chemotherapy plus a monoclonal antibody against HER2 for metastatic breast cancer that overexpresses HER2. N Engl J Med 2001;344:783–792.
ten Bokkel Huinink WW, Prove AM, Piccart M, Steward W, Tursz T, Wanders J, Franklin H, Clavel M, Verweij J, Alakl M, et al: A phase II trial with docetaxel (Taxotere) in second line treatment with chemotherapy for advanced breast cancer. A study of the EORTC Early Clinical Trials Group. Ann Oncol 1994;5:527–532.
Trudeau ME, Eisenhauer EA, Higgins BP, Letendre F, Lofters WS, Norris BD, Vandenberg TA, Delorme F, Muldal AM: Docetaxel in patients with metastatic breast cancer: a phase II study of the National Cancer Institute of Canada-Clinical Trials Group. J Clin Oncol 1996;14:422–428.
Valero V, Holmes FA, Walters RS, Theriault RL, Esparza L, Fraschini G, Fonseca GA, Bellet RE, Buzdar AU, Hortobagyi GN: Phase II trial of docetaxel: a new, highly effective antineoplastic agent in the management of patients with anthracycline-resistant metastatic breast cancer. J Clin Oncol 1995;13:2886–2894.
Yeung K, Gupta R, Haidak D, Katzen H, Greer J, Quader ML: Weekly (W) Herceptin (H, trastuzimab) and one hour Taxol (T, paclitaxel) infusion (WHT) regimen for human epidermal growth factor receptor-2 (HER2) overexpressed (+) metastatic breast cancer (MBC). Proc Am Soc Clin Oncol 2000;19:142A.

Oncology

Oncology 2001;61(suppl 2):50–57

New Combinations with Herceptin® in Metastatic Breast Cancer

Eric P. Winer Harold J. Burstein

Dana-Farber Cancer Institute, Boston, Mass., USA

Key Words

Herceptin® · Trastuzumab · HER2 · Vinorelbine · Biological therapy · Combination therapy · Metastatic breast cancer

Abstract

Preclinical data indicate that trastuzumab (Herceptin®) has the potential for synergistic or additive effects in combination with therapies including chemotherapy and hormonal agents, providing the rationale for a number of clinical trials in women with HER2-positive metastatic breast cancer. A recently reported phase II trial has demonstrated that trastuzumab plus vinorelbine is both effective (overall response rate 75%) and well tolerated, with the major side effects being typical of single-agent vinorelbine. Other combinations of trastuzumab with a variety of other chemotherapeutic and hormonal agents are also being assessed. In an effort to overcome the cardiotoxicity observed with trastuzumab plus doxorubicin in the pivotal phase III trial, combination regimens involving potentially less toxic anthracyclines such as epirubicin and liposomal formulations of doxorubicin are ongoing. In addition, trials are investigating whether trastuzumab can reverse the resistance to hormonal therapy that develops in most women with metastatic breast cancer. These and other studies will identify the regimens that produce the best outcomes with the fewest possible side effects in women with HER2-positive breast cancer.

Introduction

The humanized anti-human epidermal growth factor receptor-2 (HER2) monoclonal antibody trastuzumab (Herceptin®) is the product of a rational development process [Carter et al. 1992]. This process started with the recognition in 1987 that the HER2 proto-oncogene is involved in breast cancer development [Slamon et al. 1987, 1989] and culminated with the production of a humanized antibody targeting the oncogene in 1992 [Carter et al. 1992]. Subsequently, trastuzumab was shown to be effective in combination with chemotherapy in women with HER2-overexpressing metastatic breast cancer [Baselga et al. 1996; Baselga 1999; Baselga et al. 1999a; Cobleigh et al. 1999; Osoba and Burchmore 1999; Slamon et al. 2001]. Based on this, trastuzumab was approved for clinical use by the Food and Drug Administration in 1998 and by the European authorities in 2000.

Trastuzumab has been studied in women with HER2-positive metastatic breast cancer. The clinical benefits of trastuzumab for women with HER2-positive metastatic breast cancer were defined in a randomized study comparing chemotherapy alone versus chemotherapy plus trastuzumab. The benefits include response rates of 50% in combination with chemotherapy (paclitaxel or anthracycline plus cyclophosphamide) versus 32% with chemotherapy alone ($p < 0.0001$); improved time to progression (7.4 versus 4.6 months, $p < 0.0001$) and time to treatment failure (6.6 versus 4.5 months, $p < 0.0001$); and a significant 25% increase in survival duration (25 versus 20

KARGER

Fax +41 61 306 12 34
E-Mail karger@karger.ch
www.karger.com

0030–2414/01/0616–0050$17.50/0

Accessible online at:
www.karger.com/journals/ocl

Eric P. Winer, MD
Dana-Farber Cancer Institute
44 Binney Street, D 1214
Boston, MA 02115 (USA)
Tel. +1 617 632 3800, Fax +1 617 632 2616, E-Mail ewiner@partners.org

Table 1. Combination index (CI) scores for the effect of trastuzumab and various chemotherapeutic agents against HER2-positive breast cancer cell lines (data from Pietras et al. 1998; Konecny et al. 1999; Pegram et al. 1999b)

Effect of combination		
synergistic (CI < 1)	additive (CI = 1)	antagonistic (CI > 1)
Vinorelbine (0.34)	Doxorubicin (0.82–1.16)	Methotrexate (1.36)
Docetaxel/carboplatin (0.34)	Paclitaxel (0.91)	Gemcitabine (1.25–5.34)
Docetaxel (0.41)	Epirubicin (0.99)	5-fluorouracil (2.87)
Etoposide (0.54)	Vinblastine (1.09)	
Cyclophosphamide (0.57)		
Paclitaxel/carboplatin (0.64)		
Thiotepa (0.67)		
Cisplatin (0.56)		
Liposomal doxorubicin (0.70)		

months, $p < 0.05$) at 35 months of follow-up [Slamon et al. 2001]. Clinical activity has also been observed when trastuzumab is used as a single agent either as first-line [Vogel et al. 2000] or second- or third-line therapy for metastatic breast cancer [Cobleigh et al. 1999]. Single-agent trastuzumab is generally well tolerated and is not associated with some of the side effects seen with traditional chemotherapeutic agents [Cobleigh et al. 1999; Baselga 1999]. Most side effects are mild to moderate in severity and the more severe adverse events that have been observed, such as serious infusion-related reactions, can usually be managed using standard therapies without withdrawing trastuzumab [Cobleigh et al. 1999; Baselga 1999]. Cardiotoxicity has been observed in a small percentage of patients treated with single-agent trastuzumab or with non-anthracycline-containing combination regimens [Cobleigh et al. 1999; Seidman et al. 2001; Slamon et al. 2001; Vogel et al. 2000], but is primarily associated with concomitant anthracycline therapy. Detailed guidelines to reduce the risk of cardiotoxicity, identify changes in cardiac function while asymptomatic and manage cardiotoxicity have been formulated by European licensing authorities and include: baseline cardiac assessment including a full history and electro- or echocardiography or MUGA scan; 3-monthly cardiac monitoring during therapy, with more frequent monitoring in patients who develop asymptomatic dysfunction; use of standard medications to treat symptomatic cardiac failure if it develops; and careful risk:benefit assessment to determine whether trastuzumab withdrawal is warranted in patients who develop cardiac dysfunction.

The clinical benefits and tolerability of trastuzumab have been shown to maintain or improve patient quality of life (QoL) [Baselga et al. 1999b, Osoba et al. 1999, 2000], as would be expected based on studies indicating that tumor response is associated with improvement in specific symptoms as well as overall QoL [Seidman et al. 1995; Geels et al. 2000].

The rapid development of trastuzumab has left a number of questions that remain to be answered. Limited data are available regarding the clinical efficacy of the combination of trastuzumab with chemotherapeutic agents other than paclitaxel, anthracyclines or hormonal agents. Pegram and colleagues [1998, 1999a] have shown that the combination of trastuzumab and cisplatin has clinical efficacy; synergy has been observed with this combination in preclinical studies. Other researchers have published preliminary data regarding trastuzumab plus docetaxel [Kuzur et al. 2000, Malik et al. 2000, Nicholson et al. 2000].

Many studies to date have used preclinical models to test the interaction between trastuzumab and a wide variety of chemotherapeutic agents [Pietras et al. 1998; Pegram et al. 1999b] (table 1). These studies indicate that combinations of trastuzumab with vinorelbine, docetaxel and docetaxel plus platinum salts may have synergistic activity against breast cancer. The in vitro results shown in table 1 have been confirmed by studies using mouse xenograft models [Pietras et al. 1998; Pegram et al. 1999b]. Although the preclinical data [Shak et al. 1999] have led to the development of clinical trials, the relationship between combination index scores calculated based on preclinical observations and clinical effect has not yet been established. Therefore, while these data can be used to select the combination regimens that are most promising, the ultimate test comes with the results of clinical trials.

A number of ongoing clinical trials are examining the clinical efficacy of trastuzumab in combination with various chemotherapeutic agents. This article reviews recently reported data on the efficacy of trastuzumab plus vino-

Table 2. Reviewed studies of trastuzumab combination therapy in HER2-positive metastatic breast cancer

Study type	Details
Trastuzumab + vinorelbine	1. Single-center, phase II study of trastuzumab + vinorelbine in women who have received 0 to 2 prior regimens for metastatic disease 2. Multicenter, confirmatory phase II trial 3. Phase III trial of trastuzumab followed by trastuzumab plus vinorelbine versus trastuzumab plus vinorelbine 4. Phase III trial of trastuzumab plus vinorelbine versus trastuzumab plus taxane 5. Preoperative trial of trastuzumab plus vinorelbine for 16 weeks followed by surgery and anthracycline-based adjuvant therapy
Trastuzumab + other chemotherapy	1. Comparative phase I/II study of the cardiotoxicity of EC in HER2-negative and EC + trastuzumab in HER2-positive women 2. Comparative trial examining the cardiotoxicity of trastuzumab + FEC regimens containing 50, 75 or 100 mg/m^2 epirubicin 3. Italian trial examining the safety of trastuzumab in combination with epirubicin and docetaxel in 60 patients 4. Canadian pilot trial in which 30 patients will be treated with trastuzumab + liposomal doxorubicin
Trastuzumab + hormonal therapy	1. Anastrazole with or without trastuzumab as first-line therapy 2. First-line tamoxifen followed by tamoxifen plus trastuzumab 3. Trastuzumab plus letrozole as second-line therapy

relbine in women with HER2-overexpressing metastatic breast cancer. Ongoing studies examining the use of trastuzumab in combination with agents other than taxanes [for a review of studies of trastuzumab in combination with taxanes see Diéras et al. 2001] are also described (table 2).

A Phase II Trial of Trastuzumab plus Vinorelbine

As indicated above, preclinical studies suggest that trastuzumab may have a favorable interaction with vinorelbine. As a single agent, vinorelbine produces response rates of 16 to 50% in the metastatic breast cancer setting, depending principally on prior chemotherapy for metastatic disease [Fumoleau et al. 1995; Gasparini et al. 1994; Jones et al. 1995; Romero et al. 1994; Twelves et al. 1994; Vogel et al. 1999; Weber et al. 1995]. In these studies, weekly doses of 25 to 30 mg/m^2 were generally administered, resulting typically in a dose intensity (due to skipped doses) of 15 to 22 mg/m^2/week. Vinorelbine has a toxicity profile that suggests that it would be well tolerated with trastuzumab [Gregory and Smith, 2000]. Vinorelbine does not produce cardiac toxicity or significant nonhematologic toxicities such as alopecia, nausea and vomiting; its major side effect is myelosuppression, which is the most frequent cause of treatment delay and dose reduction. Other features that make the use of vinorelbine in combination with trastuzumab attractive include the possibility of using vinorelbine for prolonged periods and the weekly administration schedule.

Study Design

A phase II trial of weekly trastuzumab plus vinorelbine was designed with the objectives of defining the response to this regimen and of characterizing its safety profile in women with HER2-overexpressing metastatic breast cancer [Burstein et al. 2001]. To be eligible for the trial, patients had to have measurable breast cancer determined to overexpress the HER2 receptor at the 2+ or 3+ level on immunohistochemistry (IHC). Women were also required to have an Eastern Cooperative Oncology Group performance status of 0 to 2 and a left ventricular ejection fraction (LVEF) of greater than 50%.

Patients were treated with the standard dose schedule of trastuzumab (4 mg/kg intravenous (i.v.) initial dose followed by 2 mg/kg i.v. weekly) and vinorelbine 25 mg/m^2 i.v. push weekly until disease progression or toxicity. A program for modifying the dose and schedule of vinorelbine in response to myelosuppression was specified in the protocol [Burstein et al. 2001].

Patient Characteristics and Treatment Tolerability

Of the 40 patients enrolled, the majority (94%) had an ECOG performance status of 0 or 1. Other prognostically important data include the observations that 87% of patients had metastases to at least two sites, 63% of patients had liver metastases and 55% had metastases to the lung or pleura; most patients (82%) had received prior chemotherapy and approximately equal numbers of patients had and had not received prior chemotherapy for metastatic disease (52 versus 48%). No patient had received prior trastuzumab or vinorelbine therapy. Similar to the pivotal clinical trials of trastuzumab, the ratio of HER2 3+ to 2+ patients was approximately 3:1 [Burstein et al. 2001].

To evaluate the tolerability of the regimen, the necessity for vinorelbine dose adjustment and treatment-related toxicity were considered. Vinorelbine was administered at full dose in 835 of 1,044 cycles and had to be omitted completely in only 75. As expected, leukopenia and granulocytopenia were the main toxicities observed. There was no grade 3 or 4 anemia or thrombocytopenia. Grade 4 neutropenia and leukopenia developed in 10% and 5% of patients, respectively, with one patient developing febrile neutropenia. Grade 3 and 4 nonhematologic toxicity was not observed, with the exception of one episode of pancreatitis, later attributed to alcohol use. Other nonhematologic side effects were mild to moderate in nature and as expected based on the known safety profiles of trastuzumab and vinorelbine.

Cardiac function was prospectively monitored in this study. Serial cardiac assessment demonstrated that LVEF was generally maintained over the entire period of follow-up. However, three patients who were considered to have borderline cardiac function at baseline (LVEF 50 to 60%) and who had been exposed to cumulative doxorubicin doses of between 300 and 460 mg/m^2 developed asymptomatic decreases in LVEF >20% (grade 2 cardiotoxicity) or to below 50%. Therapy was withdrawn in all of these patients and LVEF stabilized or improved [Burstein et al. 2001].

Efficacy of Trastuzumab plus Vinorelbine

The overall response rate in the 40 patients enrolled in the trial was 75%, with 3 complete and 27 partial responses (table 3). Subgroup analysis showed that patients with HER2 3+ overexpression on IHC had a higher response rate than those with HER2 2+ overexpression, although the differences were not statistically significant. Response rates were similar whether or not patients had received prior chemotherapy for metastatic disease and regardless of the number of prior regimens. The type of prior chemotherapy, whether anthracyclines, taxanes or other, did not appear to affect response. However, the results suggest that patients treated with trastuzumab plus vinorelbine as first-line therapy have a longer time to treatment failure than those who received this regimen as second- or third-line therapy.

Table 3. Overall response rate of patients treated with trastuzumab plus vinorelbine. Reproduced, with permission, from Burstein et al. 2001

Type of response	Patients	Response rate, %
CR + PR	30	75
CR	3	8
PR	27	68
SD >6 months	2	5
PD	8	20

CR = Complete response; PD = progressive disease; PR = partial response; SD = stable disease.

Conclusions and Future Prospects

Trastuzumab plus vinorelbine appears to be an active and well-tolerated therapy in women with HER2-positive breast cancer. No unexpected side effects were observed and in this small study there was no indication that the combination increased the incidence or severity of known side effects associated with the individual agents. Importantly, the cardiac safety profile appeared to be reasonable and those patients who were withdrawn from therapy due to decreases in LVEF stabilized or improved. It is not known if continued treatment with this regimen in the patients who were withdrawn would have been tolerable in terms of cardiotoxicity.

The results of this trial have led to the design of further trials of trastuzumab plus vinorelbine in women with HER2-positive metastatic breast cancer. The first of these is a confirmatory phase II trial involving >10 centers in the USA. A European phase II trial involving 60 patients will also examine this combination.

Two phase III trials have been designed. The first will examine whether administering trastuzumab in combination with vinorelbine is more effective than vinorelbine alone in women who develop disease progression while receiving trastuzumab plus taxane combination therapy. The second phase III trial will randomize women to trastuzumab plus a weekly taxane or trastuzumab plus vinorelbine.

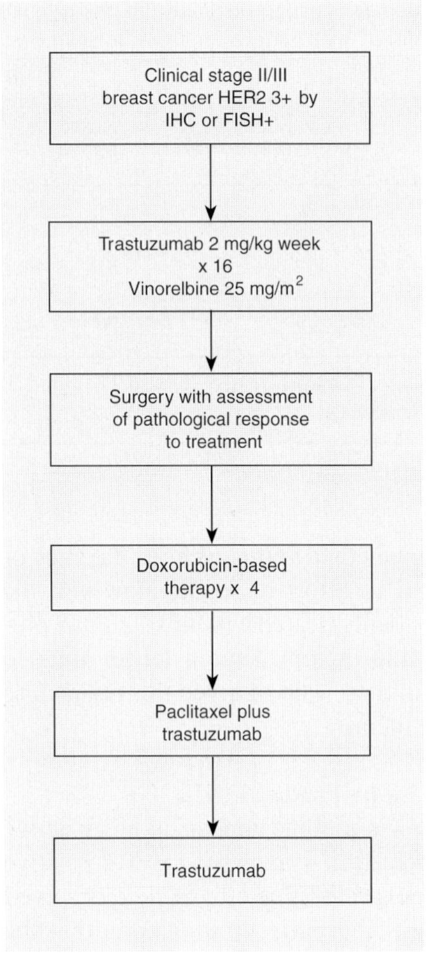

Fig. 1. Design for preoperative trial of trastuzumab plus vinorelbine in HER2-positive breast cancer (TAM = tamoxifen; XRT = radiotherapy).

At the Dana-Farber Harvard Cancer Center, a trial will open in which women with HER2 3+ or FISH-positive stage II/III breast cancer will receive 16 weeks of preoperative trastuzumab plus vinorelbine. Women will then undergo definitive surgery followed by 4 cycles of doxorubicin and additional treatment with trastuzumab plus paclitaxel (fig. 1) The primary goals of this study are to assess the pathologic complete response rate of the trastuzumab plus vinorelbine combination and to examine the tolerability of the overall regimen.

Other Trials of Trastuzumab in Combination with Chemotherapy and Hormonal Therapy

As suggested by preclinical data, various combination regimens including trastuzumab have potential clinical efficacy but have not been adequately investigated. The combination of trastuzumab and doxorubicin was shown to have a high degree of efficacy in the pivotal phase III trial, but was associated with a particularly high incidence of cardiotoxicity. Other anthracyclines, including epirubicin and liposomal forms of doxorubicin, are known to cause less cardiotoxicity and are under active investigation in combination with trastuzumab. Additional trials are investigating trastuzumab in combination with platinum analogs, the oral fluoropyrimidine capecitabine (Xeloda®), platinum analog plus taxane combinations, and hormonal therapy.

Trials of Trastuzumab in Combination with Anthracyclines Other than Doxorubicin

Epirubicin/cyclophosphamide (EC) is the standard regimen used for the treatment of metastatic breast cancer in Germany. Based on the known activity of anthracyclines in metastatic disease and evidence that epirubicin is associated with less cardiotoxicity than doxorubicin, a trial examining the combination of trastuzumab plus EC with intensive cardiac monitoring is reasonable and a German study has been initiated. Initially, 25 HER2-positive, anthracycline-naïve patients will be treated with trastuzumab plus 3-weekly EC (6 cycles at 60 mg/m^2). Cardiac safety will be closely monitored in these patients, with echocardiography being performed every 3 weeks throughout the study. Results are expected to be reported at the European Congress of Clinical Oncology in October 2001. If the cardiac outcomes are acceptable in this pilot phase, 100 HER2-positive and 100 HER2-negative women will be entered into two concurrent phase II trials. The HER2-positive women will be treated with standard-dose trastuzumab plus 3-weekly EC (4 to 6 cycles at 90 mg/m^2); HER2-negative women will be treated with 3-weekly EC alone. The cardiotoxicity observed in these two concurrent phase II trials will be compared in an effort to determine whether trastuzumab adds to the cardiotoxicity of the EC combination.

Trastuzumab in Combination with Platinum Analogs

The combination of trastuzumab with platinum analogs was one of the initial strategies tested in the early development of trastuzumab. Although these studies demonstrated that the combination was well tolerated and showed antitumor efficacy, this strategy was not pursued further because cisplatin and carboplatin are not generally used in the treatment of breast cancer. Preclinical studies have demonstrated significant synergy between trastuzumab and both carboplatin and carboplatin plus docetaxel or paclitaxel. In addition, further studies have elucidated the probable mechanism for this synergy, which involves inhibition by trastuzumab of the repair of the DNA adducts formed due to cisplatin therapy [Pietras et al. 1994, 1998].

The Breast Cancer International Research Group (BCIRG) has initiated two phase II trials involving platinum analogs in women with HER2-positive metastatic breast cancer. These trials will examine combination regimens of trastuzumab, docetaxel and cisplatin or carboplatin in North America and Europe. Preliminary data from one of the studies suggests that the side-effect profile is similar to that of docetaxel plus cisplatin in ovarian and lung cancer. If the results of the phase II trials are acceptable, the BCIRG plans to conduct large phase III trials in the adjuvant and metastatic settings. The planned adjuvant trial will enroll 2,925 HER2-positive, node-positive or high-risk node-negative patients who will be randomized to AC followed by docetaxel, AC followed by docetaxel plus trastuzumab, or docetaxel plus cisplatin/carboplatin plus trastuzumab. The metastatic breast cancer trial will compare trastuzumab plus docetaxel with trastuzumab plus docetaxel plus cisplatin/carboplatin in approximately 400 women.

Trastuzumab in Combination with Hormonal Therapy

Hormonal therapy is standard first-line treatment in women with breast cancer that expresses the estrogen (ER) and/or progesterone receptor. Clinical data obtained to date indicate that HER2 positivity may predict failure to respond to this type of treatment [De Laurentiis et al. 2000]. Furthermore, preclinical studies have demonstrated that the ER and HER2 signaling pathways may interact so that HER2 levels are increased in ER-positive cells treated with anti-estrogens such as tamoxifen [Read et al. 1990], increasing the oncogenicity of these cells and resulting in resistance to hormonal therapy [Benz et al. 1992]. Trastuzumab has been shown to reverse this apparent resistance in vitro [Witters et al. 1997; Kunisue et al. 2000]. Thus, clinical studies of trastuzumab plus hormonal agents are warranted.

Recruiting sufficient numbers of patients to such studies is made difficult because approximately 50% of all patients who are HER2 positive are hormone receptor negative. However, a number of studies are planned. In Europe, a phase II/III comparative study involving 220 patients will compare anastrazole alone with anastrazole in combination with trastuzumab as first-line therapy. Study objectives will be to determine the response rate and safety in the two arms, as well as time to progression, response duration, and one-year and overall survival. Also in Europe, a phase II trial in which trastuzumab will be added to tamoxifen at disease progression will aim to determine whether trastuzumab can modify the response to tamoxifen.

In the USA, a study to be conducted at Georgetown University, Duke University and Dana-Farber Cancer Institute will investigate the combination of trastuzumab plus letrozole as second-line therapy in metastatic breast cancer. Eligible patients will be ER-positive and HER2-positive patients who have progressed on first-line tamoxifen therapy.

Conclusions

Clinical trials involving trastuzumab have demonstrated that this novel humanized anti-HER2 monoclonal antibody is clinically effective both as a single agent and in combination with chemotherapy [Cobleigh et al. 1999; Slamon et al. 2001]. Several studies of trastuzumab-based combination therapy have focused on the efficacy of trastuzumab in combination with various dose schedules of taxanes [Kuzur et al. 2000; Nicholson et al. 2000; Seidman et al. 2001; Slamon et al. 2001]. These studies provide additional support for the benefits observed in the pivotal phase III trial. However, preclinical data indicate the potential therapeutic efficacy of trastuzumab in combination with other agents commonly used to treat breast cancer [Pietras et al. 1998; Pegram et al. 1999]. These data have provided the rationale for a number of recently reported and ongoing trials.

The combination of trastuzumab plus vinorelbine appears to be effective and well tolerated. Additional trials of this regimen are ongoing or planned, and the regimen is being used as the backbone of a trial designed to assess whether there is benefit in continuing trastuzumab after progression on a trastuzumab-containing regimen.

Other trials are assessing a variety of other chemotherapeutic and hormonal agents in combination with trastuzumab. Clinical trials examining trastuzumab in combination with less cardiotoxic anthracyclines such as epirubicin and liposomal formulations of doxorubicin are ongoing. At the same time, studies continue to investigate the underlying mechanism of the cardiotoxicity observed with trastuzumab-containing regimens. By incorporating prospective cardiac monitoring into the design of all new clinical trials, the impact of trastuzumab on cardiac function will be better characterized. It is interesting to note that the incidence of symptomatic cardiac dysfunction in recent trials has been considerably lower than that reported in the pivotal trials [Burstein et al. 2001; Seidman et al. 2001]. This difference may be due to a combination of patient selection and cardiac monitoring, allowing decreases in cardiac function to be addressed prior to the development of symptoms. These data support the guidelines for cardiac assessment and monitoring that are already widely used.

Finally, trials examining trastuzumab in combination with hormonal therapy could lead to the development of regimens that extend the efficacy of well-tolerated hormonal agents such as tamoxifen and aromatase inhibitors. The potential of using trastuzumab to reverse the resistance to hormonal therapy that develops in many women with breast cancer raises the possibility of being able to offer long-term therapy that is effective, well tolerated and maintains quality of life.

In summary, many uncertainties remain concerning the optimal use of trastuzumab in women with HER2-positive metastatic breast cancer. The large number of recently completed, ongoing, and planned studies will provide answers to many of the unresolved clinical questions.

References

Baselga J, Kerrigan M, Burchmore M, Ash M: Health-related quality of life (HRQL) in women with HER2-overexpressing metastatic breast cancer (MBC) in a phase III study of Herceptin (R) plus chemotherapy versus chemotherapy alone. Eur J Cancer 1999b;35(suppl 4):S318A.

Baselga J, Tripathy D, Mendelsohn J, Baughman S, Benz CC, Dantis L, Skarin NT, Seidman AD, Hudis CA, Moore J, Rosen PP, Twaddell T, Henderson IC, Norton L: Phase II study of weekly intravenous trastuzumab (Herceptin) in patients with HER2/*neu*-overexpressing metastatic breast cancer. Semin Oncol 1999a;26 (suppl 12):78–83.

Baselga J, Tripathy D, Mendelsohn J, Baughman S, Benz CC, Dantis L, Sklarin NT, Seidman AD, Rosen PP, Twaddell T, Henderson IC, Norton L: Phase II study of weekly intravenous recombinant humanized anti-p185^{HER2} monoclonal antibody in patients with HER2/*neu*-overexpressing metastatic breast cancer. J Clin Oncol 1996;14:737–744.

Baselga J: Safety profile of Herceptin (R) as a single agent and in combination with chemotherapy. Eur J Cancer 1999;35(suppl 4):S324A.

Benz CC, Scott GK, Sarup JC, Johnson RM, Tripathy D, Coronado E, Shepard HM, Osborne CK: Estrogen-dependent, tamoxifen-dependent tumorigenic growth of MCF-7 cells transfected with HER2/*neu*. Breast Cancer Res Treat 1992;24:85–95.

Burstein HJ, Kuter I, Campos SM, Gelman RS, Tribou L, Parker LM, Manola J, Younger J, Matulonis U, Bunnell CA, Partridge AH, Richardson PG, Clarke K, Shulman LN, Winer EP: Clinical activity of trastuzumab and vinorelbine in women with HER2-overexpressing metastatic breast cancer. J Clin Oncol 2001;19: 2722–2730.

Carter P, Presta L, Gorman CM, Ridgway JB, Henner D, Wong WL, Rowland AM, Kotts C, Carver ME, Shepard HM: Humanization of an anti-p185HER2 antibody for human cancer therapy. Proc Natl Acad Sci USA 1992;89: 4285–4289.

Cobleigh MA, Vogel CL, Tripathy D, Robert NJ, Scholl S, Fehrenbacher L, Wolter JM, Paton V, Shak S, Lieberman G, Slamon DJ: Multinational study of the efficacy and safety of humanized anti-HER2 monoclonal antibody in women who have HER2-overexpressing metastatic breast cancer that has progressed after chemotherapy for metastatic disease. J Clin Oncol 1999;17:2639–2648.

De Laurentiis M, Arpino G, Massarelli E, Carlomagno C, Ciardiello F, Tortora G, Bianco AR, De Placido S: A metanalysis of the interaction between Her2 and the response to endocrine therapy (ET) in metastatic breast cancer (MBC). Proc Am Soc Clin Oncol 2000;19: 78A.

Diéras V, Beuzeboc P, Laurence V, Pierga JY, Pouillart P: Interaction between Herceptin® and taxanes. Oncology 2001;61(suppl 2):43–49.

Fumoleau P, Delozier T, Extra JM, Canobbio L, Delgado FM, Hurteloup P: Vinorelbine (Navelbine) in the treatment of breast cancer: the European experience. Semin Oncol 1995;22(2 suppl 5):22–28.

Gasparini G, Caffo O, Barni S, Frontini L, Testolin A, Guglielmi RB, Ambrosini G: Vinorelbine is an active antiproliferative agent in pretreated advanced breast cancer patients: a phase II study. J Clin Oncol 1994;12:2094–2101.

Geels P, Eisenhauer E, Bezjak A, Zee B, Day A: Palliative effect of chemotherapy: objective tumor response is associated with symptom improvement in patients with metastatic breast cancer. J Clin Oncol 2000;18:2395–2405.

Gregory RK, Smith IE: Vinorelbine – a clinical review. Br J Cancer 2000;82:1907–1913.

Jones S, Winer E, Vogel C, Laufman L, Hutchins L, O'Rourke M, Lembersky B, Budman D, Bigley J, Hohneker J: Randomized comparison of vinorelbine and melphalan in anthracycline-refractory advanced breast cancer. J Clin Oncol 1995;13:2567–2574.

Konecny G, Pegram MD, Beryt M, Untch M, Slamon DJ: Therapeutic advantage of chemotherapy drugs in combination with Herceptin® against human breast cancer cells with HER-2/neu overexpression. Breast Cancer Res Treat 1999;57:114 (abstract 467).

Kunisue H, Kurebayashi J, Otsuki T, Tang CK, Kurosumi M, Yamamoto S, Tanaka K, Doihara H, Shimizu N, Sonoo H: Anti-HER2 antibody enhances the growth inhibitory effect of anti-oestrogen on breast cancer cells expressing both oestrogen receptors and HER2. Br J Cancer 2000;82:46–51.

Kuzur ME, Albain KS, Huntington MO, Jones SF, Hainsworth JD, Greco FA, Erland JB, Vogel CL, Burris III, HA: A phase II trial of docetaxel and Herceptin in metastatic breast cancer patients overexpressing HER-2. Proc Am Soc Clin Oncol 2000;19:131A.

Malik U, Sparano JA, Manalo J, Rajdev L, Sarta C, Hopkins U, Fineberg S: Phase II trial of weekly docetaxel (Taxotere) alone or in combination with trastuzumab (Herceptin) in patients with metastatic breast cancer. Proc Am Soc Clin Oncol 2000;19:148A.

Nicholson BP, Thor AD, Goldstein LJ, Merkel DE, Gradishar WJ, Sledge Jr GW: Weekly docetaxel (D) and rhumabher2 (H) combination therapy as first- or second-line treatment for metastatic breast cancer (MBC). Proc Am Soc Clin Oncol 2000;19:139A.

Osoba D, Burchmore M, Ash M, Tripathy D, Vogel C: Health related quality of life (HRQL) of patients with first-line, single-agent, Trastuzumab (Herceptin) for metastatic HER-2 overexpressing breast cancer. Proc Am Soc Clin Oncol 2000;19:436A.

Osoba D, Burchmore M: Health-related quality of life in women with metastatic breast cancer treated with trastuzumab (Herceptin). Semin Oncol 1999;26(suppl 12):84–88.

Pegram M, Hsu S, Lewis G, Pietras R, Beryt M, Sliwkowski M, Coombs D, Baly D, Kabbinavar F, Slamon D: Inhibitory effects of combinations of HER-2/*neu* antibody and chemotherapeutic agents used for treatment of human breast cancers. Oncogene 1999b;18:2241–2251.

Pegram MD, Lipton A, Hayes DF, Weber BL, Baselga JM, Tripathy D, Baly D, Baughman SA, Twaddell T, Glaspy JA, Slamon DJ: Phase II study of receptor-enhanced chemosensitivity using recombinant humanized anti-$p185^{HER2/neu}$ monoclonal antibody plus cisplatin in patients with HER2/*neu*-overexpressing metastatic breast cancer refractory to chemotherapy treatment. J Clin Oncol 1998;16:2659–2671.

Pegram MD, Slamon DJ: Combination therapy with trastuzumab (Herceptin) and cisplatin for chemoresistant metastatic breast cancer: evidence for receptor-enhanced chemosensitivity. Semin Oncol 1999a;26(suppl 12):89–95.

Pietras RJ, Fendly BM, Chazin VR, Pegram MD, Howell SB, Slamon DJ: Antibody to HER-2/neu receptor blocks DNA repair after cisplatin in human breast and ovarian cancer cells. Oncogene 1994;9:1829–1838.

Pietras RJ, Pegram MD, Finn RS, Maneval DA, Slamon DJ: Remission of human breast cancer xenografts on therapy with humanized monoclonal antibody to HER-2 receptor and DNA-reactive drugs. Oncogene 1998;17:2235–2249.

Read LD, Keith D, Slamon DJ, Katzenellenbogen BS: Hormonal modulation of HER2/neu protooncogene messenger ribonucleic acid and p185 protein expression in human breast cancer cell lines. Cancer Res 1990;50:3947–3951.

Romero A, Rabinovich MG, Vallejo CT, Perez JE, Rodriguez R, Cuevas MA, Machiavelli M, Lacava JA, Langhi M, Romero Acuna L: Vinorelbine as first-line chemotherapy for metastatic breast carcinoma. J Clin Oncol 1994;12:336–341.

Seidman AD, Fornier MN, Esteva FJ, Tan L, Kaptain S, Bach A, Panageas KS, Arroyo C, Valero V, Currie V, Gilewski T, Theodoulou M, Moynahan ME, Moasser M, Sklarin N, Dickler M, D'Andrea G, Cristofanilli M, Rivera E, Hortobagyi GN, Norton L, Hudis CA: Weekly trastuzumab and paclitaxel therapy for metastatic breast cancer with analysis of efficacy by HER2 immunophenotype and gene amplification. J Clin Oncol 2001;19:2587–2595.

Seidman AD, Portenoy R, Yao TJ, Lepore J, Mont EK, Kortmansky J, Onetto N, Ren L, Grechko J, Beltangady M: Quality of life in phase II trials: A study of methodology and predictive value in patients with advanced breast cancer treated with paclitaxel plus granulocyte colony stimulating factor. J Natl Cancer Inst 1995;87:1316–1322.

Shak S, for the Herceptin Multinational Investigator Study Group: Overview of the trastuzumab (Herceptin) anti-HER2 monoclonal antibody clinical program in HER2-overexpressing metastatic breast cancer. Semin Oncol 1999;26 (suppl 12):71–77.

Slamon DJ, Clark GM, Wong SG, Levin WJ, Ullrich A, McGuire WL: Human breast cancer: correlation of relapse and survival with amplification of the HER-2/*neu* oncogene. Science 1987;235:177–182.

Slamon DJ, Godolphin W, Jones LA, Holt JA, Wong SG, Keith DE, Levin WJ, Stuart SG, Udove J, Ullrich A: Studies of the HER-2/*neu* proto-oncogene in human breast and ovarian cancer. Science 1989;244:707–712.

Slamon DJ, Leyland-Jones B, Shak S, Fuchs H, Paton V, Bajamonde A, Fleming T, Eiermann W, Wolter J, Pegram M, Baselga J, Norton L: Use of chemotherapy plus a monoclonal antibody against HER2 for metastatic breast cancer that overexpresses HER2. N Engl J Med 2001;344:783–792.

Twelves CJ, Dobbs NA, Curnow A, Coleman RE, Stewart AL, Tyrrell CJ, Canney P, Rubens RD: A phase II, multicentre, UK study of vinorelbine in advanced breast cancer. Br J Cancer 1994;70:990–993.

Vogel C, Cobleigh M, Tripathy D, Harris L, Fehrenbacher L, Slamon D, Ash M, Novotny W, Stewart S, Shak S: First-line, non-hormonal, treatment of woman with HER2 overexpressing metastatic breast cancer with Herceptin (trastuzumab, humanized anti-HER2 antibody). Proc Am Soc Clin Oncol 2000;19:71A.

Vogel C, O'Rourke M, Winer E, Hochster H, Chang A, Adamkiewicz B, White R, McGuirt C: Vinorelbine as first-line chemotherapy for advanced breast cancer in women 60 years of age or older. Ann Oncol 1999;10:397–402.

Weber BL, Vogel C, Jones S, Harvey H, Hutchins L, Bigley J, Hohneker J: Intravenous vinorelbine as first-line and second-line therapy in advanced breast cancer. J Clin Oncol 1995;13:2722–30.

Witters LM, Kumar R, Chincilli VM, Lipton A: Enhanced anti-proliferative activity of the combination of tamoxifen plus HER-2-neu antibody. Breast Cancer Res Treat 1997;42:1–5.

Oncology

Oncology 2001;61(suppl 2):58–66

Retrospective Analysis of the Safety of Herceptin® Immunotherapy in Metastatic Breast Cancer

Nancy Cook-Bruns

Pharmaceuticals Development Group, F. Hoffmann-La Roche Ltd, Basel, Switzerland

Key Words

Herceptin® · Safety · Breast cancer · Cardiac safety · Infusion-related reaction · Retrospective analysis

Abstract

Approximately 25,000 patients have been treated to date with the humanized anti-HER2 monoclonal antibody, Herceptin®. This therapy has proved effective and well tolerated in patients with HER2-positive metastatic breast cancer; adverse events were generally infusion-related fever and chills of mild-to-moderate severity. Cardiotoxicity and infusion-related reactions emerged as the two main safety concerns with the use of Herceptin. Retrospective analysis revealed a higher incidence of heart failure when Herceptin was combined with anthracyclines than that expected with anthracyclines alone. Age, anthracycline exposure and cardiac risk factors were found to be predictors of cardiac adverse events. Patients experiencing cardiac dysfunction responded well to standard cardiac medication and the majority improved. Cardiac function should be monitored regularly and Herceptin should be discontinued if significant heart failure develops unless the benefits for an individual patient outweigh the risks. Of 25,000 patients, 74 (0.3%) were reported to have experienced a serious infusion-related reaction. The majority occurred during or shortly after the first infusion and were characterized by respiratory symptoms. Most patients were successfully treated; a total of 33 patients continued Herceptin therapy with no recurrence of infusion reactions. Although the benefit to risk ratio of Herceptin remains favorable, physicians must be vigilant and aggressive in managing cardiotoxicity and infusion-related reactions.

Introduction

The identification and characterization of the human epidermal growth factor receptor-2 (HER2) oncogene and its role in breast cancer [for a review, see Ross and Fletcher 1998] has led to the strategic development of a targeted immunological therapy, the humanized anti-HER2 monoclonal antibody (MAb), Herceptin® (trastuzumab) [Carter et al. 1992]. HER2 is an oncoreceptor that is overexpressed in 20 to 30% of breast cancers [Slamon et al. 1987, 1989] and is the target for Herceptin. HER2 is only expressed at low levels in normal tissue and this provides a safe therapeutic window to minimize damage to normal cells.

KARGER

Fax + 41 61 306 12 34
E-Mail karger@karger.ch
www.karger.com

0030–2414/01/0616–0058$17.50/0

Accessible online at:
www.karger.com/journals/ocl

Nancy Cook-Bruns, MD
Pharmaceuticals Development Group
F. Hoffman-La Roche Ltd
Grenzacherstrasse, CH–4070 Basel (Switzerland)
Tel. +41 61 6881180, Fax +41 61 6881520, E-Mail nancy_eileen.cook-bruns@roche.com

The current treatment of breast cancer relies on a multi-modality approach including surgery, radiation, hormone therapy, chemotherapy, supportive therapy and more recently biological therapy. In metastatic breast cancer, hormone therapy and chemotherapy are the mainstays of treatment because of the systemic nature of the disease. Surgery and radiotherapy may also be used for palliation of symptoms and to improve quality of life [Henderson et al. 1990].

The major obstacles to the success of current anticancer therapy are the presence or development of drug resistance by tumor cells and the insufficient tumor selectivity of treatment, which leads to acute or host morbidity. The many anticancer agents used in cancer chemotherapy possess either cytotoxic or cytocidal activity. However, since they are not selective, they may injure not only the cancer cells but also the normal tissues and cells of the cancer patient. The most common side effects of chemotherapy are non-specific central nervous system events (vomiting), gastrointestinal toxicity (mucositis), alopecia, myelosuppression (thrombocytopenia and leukopenia), immunosuppression, and long-term risk of inducing other malignancies [Adams 2000; Hoekman et al. 1999; Lindley et al. 1999]. Therefore, the toxicity of treatment must be balanced with the probability of gaining a meaningful response. In the hormonal treatment of breast cancer, long-term treatment with the anti-estrogen, tamoxifen, can give effective palliation in metastatic breast cancer. Although most patients treated with tamoxifen experience minimal adverse effects [Robinson et al. 1996], its estrogen-agonist activity can lead to significant side effects such as endometrial cancer and thromboembolic phenomena [Dhingra 1999]. Ocular toxicity and hepatotoxicity have also been observed but are infrequent [Robinson et al. 1996].

Biological therapy based on MAbs has many theoretical attractions and there has been a long history of research into this area [for a review, see Weiner 1999; Green et al. 2000]. One of the major expectations from the use of MAbs in cancer therapy has been that of exploiting the specificity and sensitivity of the immune system to achieve selective therapeutic effects devoid of the often severe toxicity caused by chemotherapy. Chemotherapy-associated side effects are often debilitating and have a negative impact on patient quality of life (QoL).

Until the recent approval and widespread use of trastuzumab (Herceptin) [Brenner and Adams 1999] for the treatment of breast cancer and rituximab (Rituxan®) for non-Hodgkin's lymphoma [Grillo-López et al. 1999; Leget and Czuczman 1998; Maloney and Press 1998], there had been little significant success with MAb-based anticancer therapy [Green et al. 2000]. The efficacy and tolerability of the humanized anti-HER2 MAb, Herceptin, as shown in trials where the drug was used as a single agent [Cobleigh et al. 1999; Vogel et al. 2000] or in combination with chemotherapy [Norton et al. 1999; Slamon et al. 2001], largely confirmed the expectations of immunotherapy for breast cancer. This paper discusses a retrospective analysis of the safety profile of Herceptin with a particular focus on cardiac safety and serious infusion-related reactions. Recommendations for the management of patients experiencing adverse events are also provided.

Overview of Safety of Herceptin

Clinical trials have confirmed the value of Herceptin in HER2-positive patients with metastatic breast cancer, which has led to regulatory approval of Herceptin in the USA and elsewhere [Brenner and Adams 1999]. The safety of Herceptin in cancer patients was continuously monitored from the earliest clinical studies to the post-marketing period. A global safety database held by F. Hoffmann-La Roche Ltd contains all the pharmacovigilance data relating to Herceptin. The clinical trial database has safety information on 930 patients. In addition, post-marketing surveillance data is available for more than 25,000 patients who have received Herceptin therapy since regulatory approval in the USA in September 1998 [Roche, data on file – Cook-Bruns N, McCarvil M: Cardiac task force final report. Herceptin in metastatic breast cancer. 23 June 2000].

The clinical benefit of Herceptin alone and in combination with chemotherapy in women with breast cancer was established in pivotal phase II [Cobleigh et al. 1999; Mass et al. 2000] and phase III [Mass et al. 2000; Norton et al. 1999; Slamon et al. 2001] studies, respectively. Safety data were collected in a phase II trial (study H0649g) of Herceptin as a single agent, which was conducted in 222 patients with metastatic breast cancer who had failed at least two prior chemotherapy regimens [Cobleigh et al. 1999] and in the phase III combination trial of Herceptin plus chemotherapy (study H0648g) [Norton et al. 1999; Slamon et al. 2001]. Both trials indicated that Herceptin is generally well tolerated and is associated with side effects that are generally mild to moderate. In the pivotal phase II trial, approximately 40% of patients experienced fever and chills that were associated primarily with the first infusion. Other less frequently occurring side effects included nausea, pain, headache and dizziness. The most clinically significant adverse events were signs and symptoms of cardiac dysfunction. It is noteworthy that the adverse events typically observed following cytotoxic chemotherapy, such as myelosuppression, mucositis and alopecia, were rarely observed with Herceptin monotherapy. In the phase III trial, conducted in 469 women with HER2-positive metastatic breast cancer, the efficacy and safety of first-line Herceptin plus chemotherapy regimens (paclitaxel or anthracycline plus cyclophosphamide) was compared with chemotherapy alone [Norton et al. 1999; Slamon et al. 2001]. As with single-agent therapy, infusion-related signs and symptoms such as chills and fevers were the most common types of events, with a higher incidence in Herceptin plus chemotherapy treated patients than in the parallel chemotherapy alone groups. Furthermore, there was an increased rate of infections, mainly due to respiratory and catheter-related infections in the Herceptin plus chemotherapy treatment group compared with those patients who received chemotherapy alone. Although respiratory infections were of minor clinical significance, there may be an increased risk of catheter infections with Herceptin because of the increased catheter handling involved with weekly infusions.

In addition, four cases of acute leukemia or myelodysplastic syndrome were identified in the patient subgroup receiving concomitant Herceptin plus chemotherapy. Each of the patients had risk factors for leukemia with prior chemotherapy exposure and/or prior radiotherapy exposure. The development of leukemia in patients with metastatic breast cancer treated with chemotherapy has been well described in the literature [Pegram et al. 1998]. Herceptin appears to be non-immunogenic; only one of 903 patients evaluated in an integrated safety database developed neutralizing antibodies to Herceptin. Clinically, the patient had no signs or symptoms of allergy while receiving Herceptin and discontinued the study after nine infusions because of disease progression.

In summary, the pivotal trials showed that Herceptin therapy is generally well tolerated with mild-to-moderate side effects. Significantly, the side-effect profile of Herceptin differs from that associated with chemotherapy in that there is a low incidence of side effects such as myelosuppression, mucositis and alopecia. However, cardiotoxicity and infusion-related reactions have emerged as the two main safety concerns with the use of Herceptin in patients with metastatic breast cancer, as reviewed in detail below.

Cardiac Safety

During pivotal clinical trials to assess the efficacy and safety of Herceptin, a signal of cardiac toxicity was noted. As a result, a Cardiac Review and Evaluation Committee (CREC) was set up to monitor cardiac adverse events. The unexpected cardiac toxicity observed in the pivotal trials of Herceptin could not have been predicted based on the mechanism of action of the antibody or from safety data obtained in early Herceptin trials. A retrospective evaluation of all cases of cardiac dysfunction to December 1997 was performed by the CREC and its report was included in the United States (US) and European Union (EU) regulatory submissions [Roche, data on file – Summary and analysis of Cardiac Review and Evaluation Committee (CREC) findings. Application for marketing authorization application (MAA) for HERCEPTIN, part I: Summary of the dossier section I.C.3.6 Ref. 0008.]. The events identified as having a higher incidence under Herceptin treatment, in particular in combination with anthracycline/cyclophosphamide (AC), were events related to heart failure and were typical of anthracycline-induced cardiotoxicity.

A second evaluation of cardiac adverse events with Herceptin was requested by the European Committee for Proprietary Medicinal Products (CPMP) as part of the European marketing authorization application. A Cardiac Task Force, comprised of F. Hoffmann La-Roche Ltd physicians and an external advisory board of cardiologists, was set up for this purpose. The objective of the re-analysis was to confirm the relative incidence of anthracycline-typical cardiac events as well as to determine the incidence of other cardiac events.

The re-analysis included newly reported adverse events from all trials until March 2000 and follow-up data that had not been included in the CREC evaluation, and a distinction was made between asymptomatic drop in left ventricular ejection fraction (LVEF) and symptomatic heart failure. From the pivotal clinical trials, the clinical research forms (CRFs) of the 41 patients who were identified as having experienced an event were reviewed by F. Hoffmann La-Roche Ltd physicians and a medical assessment was made [Roche, data on file – Cook-Bruns N, McCarvil M: Cardiac task force final report. Herceptin in metastatic breast cancer. 23 June 2000].

Incidence of Cardiac Events

The incidence of cardiac dysfunction, which was the most clinically significant adverse event in both pivotal

Table 1. An overview of the incidence of cardiac adverse events in the pivotal trials

	Combination study H0648g				Monotherapy study H0649g (n = 213)
	P + H (n = 91)	P (n = 95)	AC + H (n = 143)	AC (n = 135)	
AC, mg/m^2					
Median (50%)	245	238	347	346	316
3Q (75%)	320	301	376	359	473
Incidence CHF, %	8.8–11.0	1.0–4.0	26.0–28.0	6.0–9.6	6.0–8.8

Incidence of heart failure: retrospective evaluation H0648 g, H0649g.
Roche cardiac update: cut-off March 1999.

trials, is summarized in table 1. For the purpose of the analysis, cardiac adverse events were grouped under 'symptomatic heart failure' (excluding drop in LVEF), 'definitive cardiac diagnosis other than heart failure' or 'event unevaluable as to etiology'. Thus, symptomatic heart failure has been separated from asymptomatic drop in ejection fraction. This is important because the prognostic significance of asymptomatic drops in LVEF, especially in patients with metastatic breast cancer, is not fully elucidated [Brockstein et al. 2000].

The rate of symptomatic heart failure (anthracycline-typical) in patients who received monotherapy in the pivotal phase II trial ranged from 6.0 to 8.5%, the higher rate being reported in the second retrospective evaluation due to the different criteria used to define cardiac dysfunction. Notably, all but one of the patients with heart failure had received prior anthracyclines. The doses of anthracycline received were particularly high in the monotherapy study, which explains the higher rate of cardiotoxicity.

In the pivotal phase III combination trial, the rate of symptomatic heart failure for Herceptin in combination with paclitaxel was 8.8% whereas the rate of cardiac dysfunction was 11.0% (the combined rate of symptomatic heart failure events and asymptomatic drops in left ventricular ejection fraction). Although these rates are not significantly different ($p = 0.204$) from that for paclitaxel alone where the rate of symptomatic heart failure was 4% (table 1), comparisons are difficult here as there was no measurement of left ventricular ejection fraction in the paclitaxel arm of the trial. It is noteworthy that almost all the patients in the paclitaxel and paclitaxel plus Herceptin arms (98%) had received previous anthracycline treatment for metastatic breast cancer. There was, however, a statistically significant ($p < 0.001$) increase in the incidence of congestive heart failure with Herceptin plus AC relative to AC alone (range 26 to 28% versus range 6.0 to 9.6%). Notably, the increased incidence of symptomatic cardiotoxicity was typical of anthracycline-induced cardiotoxicity and was characterized by shortness of breath, pulmonary and peripheral edema, and cardiomegaly. Importantly, the incidence of other cardiac events not typical of anthracycline-induced cytotoxicity was not significantly increased under Herceptin treatment in combination with either anthracycline or paclitaxel when compared with either chemotherapy alone.

Management of Cardiac Dysfunction

The majority of patients who experienced cardiac dysfunction showed improvement with conservative standard treatment for cardiac dysfunction (angiotensin-converting enzyme [ACE] inhibitors, diuretics and cardiac glycosides). As illustrated in figure 1, there was no obvious difference in the outcome of patients who continued Herceptin therapy compared with those who withdrew from therapy. Of the 41 patients with symptomatic heart failure in the pivotal studies, 28 continued Herceptin therapy and 13 withdrew. Furthermore, permanent disability or persistent deterioration in cardiac status was unusual. In the entire clinical database, only seven deaths were attributed at least partly to a cardiac event. There were five spontaneous reports of death and 25 deaths occurred in clinical trials during the post-approval period up to March 2000. In the clinical trial reports, other than the above seven cases of death, the deaths were attributed to other causes, mainly disease progression.

Risk Factors for Cardiotoxicity

The evidence so far indicates that cardiotoxicity is mainly related to prior or concomitant anthracycline exposure and is unlikely to be induced by Herceptin alone. Anthracyclines are associated with a high incidence

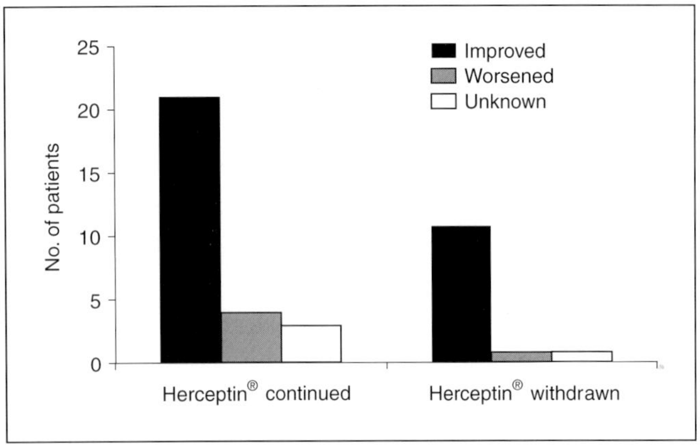

Fig. 1. Summary of outcome in patients with heart failure in the pivotal studies. Heart failure improved whether Herceptin was continued or withdrawn.

of cardiotoxicity [Ewer et al. 1999, Lefrak et al. 1973]. Prior anthracycline exposure was a major common factor in patients who developed cardiac failure during combination treatment. In the paclitaxel groups in study H0648g, all patients with heart failure events had been previously exposed to anthracyclines at cumulative doses ranging from approximately 100 to 1,200 mg/m^2. No obvious threshold of prior exposure was identified. Congestive heart failure and a decrease in cardiac systolic function are the primary clinical characteristics of anthracycline toxic effects on the heart.

A multivariate analysis was performed on the pivotal phase III trial data. This indicated that prior anthracycline exposure and other known risk factors for cardiac dysfunction such as age ≥ 50 years, New York Heart Association (NYHA) class ≥ 2 and hyperlipidemia predicted for cardiac-related adverse events in all patients in the paclitaxel arms, irrespective of Herceptin treatment. After the data were adjusted for these predictive factors, Herceptin treatment was still not found to be a significant risk factor for cardiac events in the paclitaxel arms of the study ($p = 0.185$). However, adjusting the data in the AC arms for significant risk factors for cardiac dysfunction revealed a trend showing an effect of Herceptin treatment ($p = 0.091$). This result is consistent with the increased incidence in cardiac failure observed in the Herceptin plus AC subgroup relative to the AC alone subgroup.

Anthracycline-Naïve Patients

The incidence of heart failure in anthracycline-naïve patients was determined by analyzing the cardiac safety data from the pivotal phase II single-agent Herceptin trial and a phase II trial (H0650g) of single-agent Herceptin as first-line therapy [Vogel et al. 2000]. Significantly, patients who had not received prior anthracycline therapy showed a significantly lower level of cardiotoxicity. Of the 84 anthracycline-naïve patients in these clinical trials, only three (4%) developed heart failure. All three patients were elderly, had a history of cardiac disease and improved with standard treatment for heart failure. These findings support that Herceptin has no inherent cardiotoxicity and does not directly lead to cardiac failure.

Mechanism of Cardiotoxicity

A number of hypotheses have been proposed to explain the observed cardiotoxicity. It is noteworthy that there is currently no strong evidence to suggest a direct cardiotoxic effect from Herceptin treatment alone. Preclinical studies of Herceptin did not show an effect on cardiac tissues in animals. An increased level of cardiac dysfunction was therefore not anticipated in the pivotal trials. Furthermore, the HER2 receptor is not overexpressed in normal human cardiac myocytes. The effects of Herceptin on the cardiac muscle and the mechanisms underlying the increased cardiotoxicity observed in combination with anthracyclines in the pivotal trials are not understood. Anthracyclines are known to induce cardiomyopathy [Singal and Iliskovic 1998]. However, it is possible that Herceptin may interfere with growth and repair after anthracycline-induced damage. Research is ongoing into the growth factor receptor family and their importance in the myocyte survival pathways. HER2 receptors seem to be cardioprotective because they mediate the activation of important cardiac survival pathways. Furthermore, the GP130 system is a protective factor in the myocyte and prevents apoptosis of the cardiac cells, and evidence suggests that it may interact with the HER2 receptor. Studies are continuing to investigate the proposed mechanisms and to develop new hypotheses [Feldman et al. 2000]. In addition, a number of clinical trials are underway to examine cardiac safety with Herceptin in combination with anthracyclines such as epirubicin and liposomal doxorubicin, which are associated with a lower incidence of cardiotoxicity than doxorubicin.

Recommendations for Detection and Management of Cardiac Dysfunction

Based on current knowledge, the following guidelines are proposed for cardiac evaluation and management of patients receiving Herceptin. The recommendations were developed in association with a panel of cardiology experts.

- In patients with symptomatic heart failure, a history of hypertension or documented coronary artery disease (CAD), a careful risk:benefit assessment should be made before deciding to treat with Herceptin;
- Cardiac function should be assessed at baseline using eletrocardiography (ECG), echocardiography or multigated radionuclide angiography (MUGA) scan and further monitored during treatment (e.g., every 3 months);
- Cardiac function should be monitored regularly in order to detect cardiac adverse events early;
- If cardiac failure develops during Herceptin therapy, it should be treated with the standard medication;
- Patients who develop asymptomatic cardiac dysfunction may benefit from more frequent monitoring (e.g. every 6 to 8 weeks). If decrease in LVEF persists, the physician should consider discontinuing therapy if there has been no clinical benefit from Herceptin;
- In patients who develop clinically significant heart failure, Herceptin should be discontinued unless the benefits for an individual patient are deemed to outweigh the risks.

Risk:Benefit Assessment

Taken together, the data obtained by retrospective analysis of the cardiac safety data and the pivotal trials data indicate that Herceptin has a favorable risk:benefit ratio and can, therefore, be used safely with appropriate monitoring of cardiac dysfunction. Notably, the majority of patients who developed symptomatic heart failure in the clinical trials improved with standard medical management, and the outcome of these patients was similar whether Herceptin therapy was continued or withdrawn. An analysis of the pivotal trial data also showed that time to unfavorable clinical outcome (death, progressive disease or heart failure) was significantly longer in the Herceptin treatment groups than in the control groups. Thus, it appears that patients experiencing heart failure continued to benefit from Herceptin therapy.

Serious Infusion-Related Reactions

As indicated above, mild-to-moderate infusion reactions were found to be common in the pivotal trials. These were, however, transient and could be managed by interrupting the infusion or by the use of analgesics or other medications as appropriate. Reports of serious infusion-related events have been rare although there have been a small number of fatalities. A review of the causes of death suggested that dyspnea at rest in patients with advanced breast cancer is a predisposing factor to fatal outcome. Post-marketing surveillance data, until March 2000, includes 74 reports worldwide of serious infusion-related events from the 25,000 patients treated with Herceptin. Most patients had a favorable outcome: 65 of the 74 patients responded well to supportive treatment. Of the 39 patients who are known to have been rechallenged following withdrawal of Herceptin infusion, 33 were rechallenged successfully and then continued to receive treatment with Herceptin. Nine patients died, an approximate reported incidence of 0.04%. There were a further six deaths of unclear etiology.

The 74 patients who experienced serious infusion-related reactions presented with various symptoms as summarized in table 2. Most of the patients complained of respiratory symptoms (65%) or of chills/rigors (32%). Reduced oxygen saturation was reported in 15% and hypotension and fever in 14% of patients. The nine (12%) patients who experienced respiratory failure died. Most patients experienced the serious infusion-related reactions with the first infusion and not with subsequent infusions (fig. 2). It is important to note that most of the serious infusion-related reactions occurred within 2 h after the start of the first infusion (fig. 3). Some patients developed symptoms (e.g., bronchospasm and dyspnea) 15 to 20 min after the beginning of the infusion. Very few patients experienced a reaction after the end of the infusion. However, two patients died suddenly the day after the infusion.

A review of the nine patients who died following an infusion-related reaction revealed that all these patients had pre-existing, severe, malignancy-related respiratory distress. Six of the nine patients had symptomatic and severe respiratory insufficiency secondary to the underlying malignancy, and four of these patients were receiving supplemental oxygen when the first Herceptin infusion was administered. One patient with superior vena caval thrombosis had a bacterial pneumonia and one patient with liver failure also had pneumonia. One patient who had pulmonary and pleural metastases died due to sinus bradycardia after receiving a paclitaxel and Herceptin infusion; sinus bradycardia is a known side effect of paclitaxel and thus may account for the fatal reaction.

As a result of the fatal infusion-related reactions, a warning was issued in the form of a 'Dear doctor' letter.

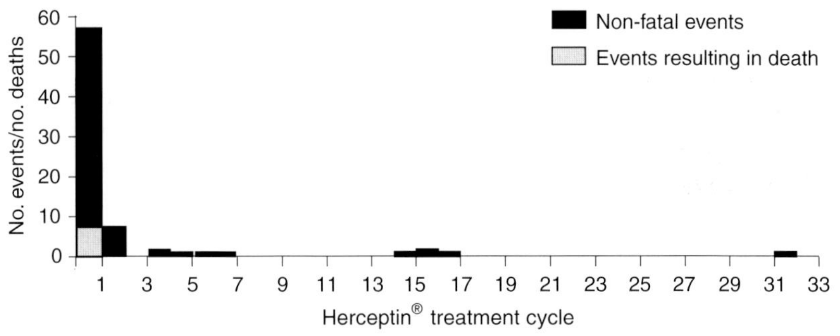

Fig. 2. Most serious infusion-related reactions occur with the first infusion.

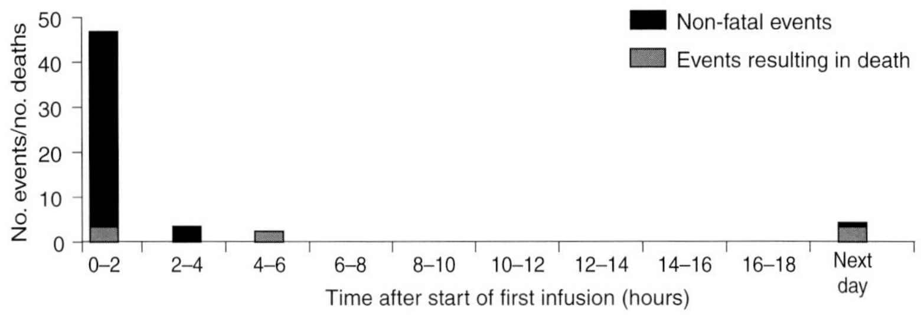

Fig. 3. Most serious infusion-related reactions occur within 2 h of the start of the first infusion.

Table 2. Serious infusion-related reactions

	Cut-off	
	30 November 1999 (6 months)	31 March 2000 (4 months)
Cumulative serious infusion reactions	54	74
Deaths	6	9
Symptoms of serious infusion reactions		
Patients with respiratory symptoms		48 (65%)
Chills or rigors		24 (32%)
Reduced O_2sat		11 (15%)
Hypotension		10 (14%)
Bradycardia		2 (3%)
Tachycardia		8 (11%)
Swelling		4 (5%)
Fever		10 (14%)
Nausea and vomiting		8 (11%)
Rash, itching, hives		6 (8%)
Respiratory failure		9 (12%)

This letter communicated that patients with severe dyspnea at rest or those requiring supplementary oxygen therapy due to complications of advanced malignancy may be at increased risk of fatal infusion reactions.

Recommendations for Detecting and Managing Serious Infusion-Related Reactions

It is recommended that patients should be observed for signs of infusion-related symptoms, especially during the first infusion. Mild symptoms may be treated with an analgesic, an antipyretic such as meperedine or paracetamol, or an antihistamine such as diphenhydramine. In addition, the serious reactions have been successfully managed with withdrawal of Herceptin and with supportive therapy such as oxygen, beta antagonists and corticosteroids.

Conclusions

A retrospective analysis has been performed on the cumulative safety data available for the anti-HER2 monoclonal antibody, Herceptin. This analysis shows that Herceptin is generally well tolerated and has a very favorable adverse-event profile compared with that of other chemotherapeutic agents. In addition, Herceptin does not usually increase the side effects expected with chemotherapy alone. The most frequent side effects are mild-to-moderate, transient effects such as fever and chills, which can be more of an inconvenience than an adverse effect. Importantly, Herceptin is not associated with the typical chemotherapy-induced complications, such as hair loss and myelosuppression.

The main serious adverse event associated with Herceptin therapy is cardiac dysfunction. Although current data indicate that Herceptin can lead to cardiac dysfunction, especially in combination with anthracyclines, this adverse event is reversible with standard medical management in the majority of affected patients. Moreover, with medical management there is rarely any deterioration in cardiac function with further Herceptin therapy. Ongoing studies should determine the nature of the cardiotoxicity seen with Herceptin therapy. No conclusive evidence is available to suggest that Herceptin alone is the cause of cardiac dysfunction. Serious infusion-related reactions have also been identified as clinically relevant adverse events. However, they occur mainly in patients who are predisposed or at risk, are infrequent and occur primarily within 2 h of the start of the first infusion. Although the risk:benefit ratio of Herceptin therapy remains favorable, it is recommended that physicians monitor patients carefully and be aggressive in treating infusion-related reactions. Overall, the significant efficacy of Herceptin in breast cancer coupled with its favorable safety profile make this novel biological therapy an important and attractive therapeutic option for HER2-positive breast cancer patients.

References

Adams VR: Adverse events associated with chemotherapy for common cancers. Pharmacotherapy 2000;20:S96–S103.

Brenner TL, Adams VR: First MAb approved for the treatment of metastatic breast cancer. J Am Pharm Assoc 1999;39:236–238.

Brockstein BE, Smiley C, Al-Sadir J, Williams SF: Cardiac and pulmonary toxicity in patients undergoing high dose chemotherapy for lymphoma and breast cancer: prognostic factors. Bone Marrow Transplant 2000;25:885–894.

Carter P, Presta L, Gorman CM, Ridgway JB, Henner D, Wong WL, Rowland AM, Kotts C, Carver ME, Shepard HM: Humanization of the anti-p185HER2 antibody for human cancer therapy. Proc Natl Acad Sci USA 1992;89: 4285–4289.

Cobleigh MA, Vogel CL, Tripothy D, Robert NJ, Scholl S, Fehrenbacher L, Wolter JM, Paton V, Shak S, Lieberman G, Slamon DJ: Multinational study of the efficacy and safety of humanized anti-HER2 monoclonal antibody in women who have HER2-overexpressing metastatic breast cancer that has progressed after chemotherapy for metastatic disease. J Clin Oncol 1999;17:2639–2648.

Dhingra K: Antiestrogens – tamoxifen, SERMS and beyond. Invest New Drugs 1999;17:285–311.

Ewer MS, Gibbs HR, Swafford J, Benjamin RS: Cardiotoxicity in patients receiving Trastuzumab (Herceptin): primary toxicity, synergistic or sequential stress, or surveillance artefact? Semin Oncol 1999;26:96–101.

Feldman AM, Lorell BH, Reis SE: Trastuzumab in the treatment of metastatic breast cancer: anticancer therapy versus cardiotoxicity. Circulation 2000;102:272–274.

Green MC, Murray JL, Hortobagyi GN: Monoclonal antibody therapy for solid tumors. Cancer Treat Rev 2000;26:269–286.

Grillo-López AJ, White CA, Varns C, Shen D, Wei A, McClure A, Ballaire BK: Overview of the clinical development of rituximab: first monoclonal antibody approved for the treatment of lymphoma. Semin Oncol 1999;26;66–73.

Henderson IC, Garber JE, Breitmeyer JB, Hayes DF, Harris JR: Comprehensive management of disseminated breast cancer. Cancer 1990;66: 1439–1448.

Hoekman K, van der Vijgh WJ, Vermorken JB: Clinical and preclinical modulation of chemotherapy-induced toxicity in patients with cancer. Drugs 1999;57:133–155.

Lefrak E, Pitha J, Rosenheim S, Gottlieb JA: A clinicopathological analysis of Adriamycin cardiotoxicity. Cancer 1973;32:302–314.

Leget GA, Czuczman MS: Use of rituximab, the new FDA-approved antibody. Curr Opin Oncol 1998;10:548–551.

Lindley C, McCune JS, Thomason TE, Lauder D, Sauls A, Adkins S, Sawyer WT: Perception of chemotherapy side effects cancer versus noncancer patients. Cancer Practice 1999;7:59–65.

Maloney DG, Press OW: Newer treatments for non-Hodgkin's lymphoma: monoclonal antibodies. Oncology 1998;12:63–76.

Mass RD, Sanders C, Charlene K, Johnson L, Everett T, Anderson S: The concordance between the clinical trials assay (CTA) and fluorescence in situ hybridization (FISH) in the Herceptin pivotal trials. Proc Am Soc Clin Oncol 2000; 19:75A.

Norton L, Slamon D, Leyland-Jones B, Wolter J, Fleming T, Eirmann W, Baselga J, Mendelsohn J, Bajamonde A, Ash M, Shak S: Overall survival (OS) advantage to simultaneous chemotherapy (CRx) plus the humanized anti-HER2 monoclonal antibody Herceptin (H) in HER2-overexpressing (HER2+) metastatic breast cancer (MBC). Proc Am Soc Clin Oncol 1999;18:127A.

Pegram MD, Lipton A, Hayes DF, Weber BL, Baselga JM, Tripathy D, Baly D, Baughman SA, Twaddell T, Glaspy JA, Slamon DJ: Phase II study of receptor-enhanced chemosensitivity using recombinant humanized anti-p185HER2/neu monoclonal antibody plus cisplatin in patients with HER2/neu-over-expressing metastatic breast cancer refractory to chemotherapy treatment. J Clin Oncol 1998;16:2659–2671.

Robinson E, Kimmick GG, Musa HB: Tamoxifen in postmenopausal women a safety perspective. Drugs Aging 1996;8:329–337.

Ross JS, Fletcher JA: The HER-2/neu oncogene in breast cancer: prognostic factor, predictive factor, and target for therapy. Stem Cells 1998;16:413–428.

Singal PK, Iliskovic N: Doxorubicin-induced cardiomyopathy. N Engl J Med 1998;339:900–905.

Slamon DJ, Clark GM, Wong SG Levin WJ, Ullrich A, McGuire WL: Human breast cancer: correlation of relapse and survival with amplification of the HER-2/*neu* oncogene. Science 1987;235:177–182.

Slamon DJ, Godolphin W, Jones LA, Holt JA, Wong SG, Keith DE, Levin WJ, Stuart SG, Udove J, Ullrich A, Press MF: Studies of the HER2/*neu* proto-oncogene in human breast and ovarian cancer. Science 1989;244:707–712.

Slamon D, Leyland-Jones B, Shak S, Paton V, Bajamonde A, Fleming T, Eiermann W, Wolter J, Baselga J, Norton L: Use of chemotherapy plus a monoclonal antibody against HER2 for metastatic breast cancer that overexpresses HER2. N Engl J Med 2001;344:783–792.

Vogel C, Cobleigh M, Tripathy D, Harris L, Fehrenbacher L, Slamon D, Ash M, Novotny W, Stewart S, Shak S: First-line, non-hormonal, treatment of women with HER2 overexpressing metastatic breast cancer with Herceptin (trastuzumab, humanized anti-HER2 antibody). Proc Am Soc Clin Oncol 2000;19:71A.

Weiner LM: An overview of monoclonal antibody therapy of cancer. Semin Oncol 1999;26:41–50.

Oncology

Oncology 2001;61(suppl 2):67–72

HER2 as a Prognostic Factor in Breast Cancer

Sylvie Ménard Stefania Fortis Fabio Castiglioni Roberto Agresti
Andrea Balsari

Istituto Nazionale Tumori and Institute of Pathology, University of Milan, Milan, Italy

Key Words
HER2 · Prognostic factor · Tumor phenotype · Infiltrating ductal carcinoma · Ductal carcinoma in situ · Lymphoid infiltration · Atypical ductal hyperplasia

Abstract
HER2 amplification/overexpression is a marker of poor prognosis in breast cancer. The prognostic impact of HER2 positivity is lower in node-negative compared with node-positive women. The only significant, independent prognostic factors in breast cancer are node status, HER2 status and menopausal status. HER2-positive tumors also contain p53 abnormalities, tend to be hormone receptor and bcl-2 negative, have lymphoid infiltration (LI) and a high mitotic index. Patients with LI who are HER2 positive have a better prognosis than those who are HER2 negative, whereas HER2-positive patients without LI have a significantly worse prognosis than HER2-negative patients. Morphological and biological alterations appear to identify two categories of breast tumor. Two hypotheses may explain the progression to two tumor types: (1) atypical ductal hyperplasia (ADH) is a precursor of ductal carcinoma in situ (DCIS), which is a precursor of invasive ductal carcinoma (IDC); or (2) ADH is a precursor of HER2-negative IDC whereas DCIS is a precursor of HER2-positive IDC. The second theory fits well with two breast cancer subsets and the characteristics of ADH and DCIS. The first type of IDC occurs in older patients, progresses slowly due to estrogen dependency but is aggressive long term. The other type progresses rapidly, is HER2 positive and is more likely to occur in young patients.

Introduction

Risk evaluation assessment to obtain prognoses for patients presenting with breast cancer is typically performed by examining a number of well-recognized pathologic features such as tumor type, histologic grade, tumor size and nodal involvement. This enables a physician to establish whether patients have indolent or aggressive disease and to select the appropriate treatment. Overall, the most reliable, independent marker of poor prognosis in breast cancer patients is the presence of metastases in regional lymph nodes [Hynes and Stern 1994]. However, combination of individual factors such as tumor grade and lymph node status carries greater predictive weight for prognosis than any individual factor. In addition to the above risk factors, estrogen-receptor (ER) and progesterone-receptor (PgR) status have been shown to have prognostic value in breast cancer, although the importance of hormone-receptor status lies more as a predictor of response to endocrine therapy [Clark et al. 1983;

KARGER
Fax +41 61 306 12 34
E-Mail karger@karger.ch
www.karger.com

0030–2414/01/0616–0067$17.50/0

Accessible online at:
www.karger.com/journals/ocl

Sylvie Ménard, MD
Molecular Targeting Unit, Department of Experimental Oncology
Istituto Nazionale Tumori, Via Venezian 1
I–20133 Milan (Italy)
Tel. +39 02 2390 571, Fax +39 02 2362 692, E-Mail menard@istitutotumori.mi.it

Thorpe 1988]. Thus, breast cancer patients whose tumors overexpress these receptors are hormone responsive and therefore have a significantly better prognosis compared with patients whose tumors are ER/PgR negative [Thorpe 1988].

In recent times, a number of molecular markers have been identified that may have prognostic value. Of these, the human epidermal growth factor receptor-2 (HER2; also known as c-*erb*B-2 or HER2/*neu*) is one of the most promising. The HER2 protein is a 185-kD transmembrane glycoprotein and a member of the HER family of growth factor receptors [Coussens et al. 1985; Hynes and Stern 1994; for a review, see Yarden 2001]. HER2 heterodimerizes with other members of the HER family and participates in signal transduction cascades [Graus-Porta et al. 1997]. The HER2 protein is involved in the regulation of normal breast growth and development [DiAugustine and Richards 1997; Normanno and Ciardiello 1997]. HER2 gene amplification/protein overexpression has been detected in 20 to 30% of human breast carcinomas and studies have indicated that HER2 amplification/overexpression plays a role in malignant transformation and tumorigenesis [Di Fiore et al. 1987; Hudziak et al. 1987; Slamon et al. 1987, 1989]. HER2 overexpression was first reported in ductal carcinoma in situ (DCIS) breast cancer by van de Vijver et al. [1988] and was associated with the comedo carcinoma variant. Several groups subsequently reported the presence of HER2 abnormalities in high-grade and comedo DCIS [for a review, see Allred et al. 1992a; Ross and Fletcher 1998].

This paper examines the relationship between HER2 positivity and morphological and biological alterations and how they impact on prognosis in breast cancer. Two hypotheses regarding the progression of precursor lesions to form two distinct subsets of breast cancer are also presented and discussed.

HER2 as a Prognostic Factor: Node-Positive versus Node-Negative Disease

The clinical utility of HER2 as a predictor of poor prognosis has received considerable attention [for a review, see Ross and Fletcher 1998]. Slamon and colleagues [1987] were the first to demonstrate that HER2 amplification/overexpression independently predicts for more aggressive disease behavior and a reduced overall and disease-free survival in node-positive patients. Subsequently, many studies have evaluated the prognostic significance of HER2 overexpression in breast cancer. Retrospective, multivariate analysis of data from 47 studies involving more than 15,000 patients confirmed that, in the majority (60%) of studies and the majority (67%) of patients, a HER2-positive status was an independent predictor of a worse prognosis in node-positive patients [Ross and Fletcher 1998].

Studies evaluating HER2 status and prognosis in node-negative patients, however, have yielded conflicting results [for a review, see Ross and Fletcher 1998]. The reliability and comparability of these studies are limited by a number of factors, including evaluation of small numbers of patients, inconsistencies in post-surgical treatment and in the methods used for the assessment of HER2 status. Although node-negative patients generally have a better prognosis following surgery than node-positive patients, approximately one-third of node-negative patients will eventually develop metastatic disease [Allred et al. 1992b]. Therefore, it is important to identify those node-negative patients at higher risk of progressing to metastatic disease who could benefit from clinical intervention with an appropriate adjuvant therapy.

A retrospective analysis of 1,200 primary breast cancer samples from patients who were treated surgically but received no systemic adjuvant therapy, as it was not available at the time of study, confirmed that HER2 status has a strong impact on the survival of node-positive patients (fig. 1). These data show that the 5-year survival rate is approximately 20% less for HER2-positive, node-positive women than HER2-negative, node-positive women. Interestingly, HER2 status only impacts on survival during the first 4–5 years following surgery. After this period, survival in patients with HER2-positive tumors parallels that of patients with HER2-negative tumors. This study also shows that the prognostic significance of HER2 is much lower in node-negative patients relative to node-positive patients, with HER2 positivity associated with only a 5% reduction in survival.

Rilke and colleagues [1991] examined the relationship of HER2 with a range of pathological, clinical, and biological factors known or suggested to have an impact on breast cancer prognosis. In total, the archived, surgical specimens from 2,000 breast cancer patients were systematically evaluated for 18 clinicopathologic parameters. As expected, the two most significant, individual, prognostic factors were lymph node status and tumor size. Other single factors (in decreasing order of significance) with a significant impact on survival were mitotic index, tumor grade, menopausal status, HER2 status and age. However, multifactorial analysis using a Cox regression model revealed that only lymph node involvement (p =

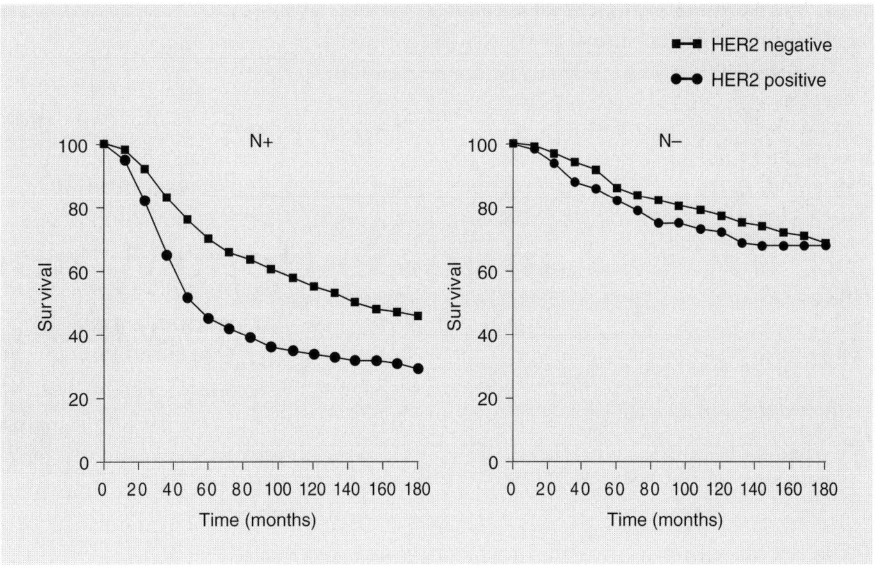

Fig. 1. Survival in relation to tumor HER2 status in patients with primary breast cancer treated surgically, with no systemic adjuvant therapy.

0.000007), HER2 protein overexpression (p = 0.0007) and menopausal status (p = 0.02) have a statistically significant, independent impact on survival. This result was surprising because although menopausal status would be expected to substitute for age and node status for tumor size, the substitution of all other biological parameters by HER2 status is unexpected. However, tumors that overexpress HER2 also contain p53 abnormalities and tend to be hormone receptor and bcl-2 negative, and have lymphoid infiltration (LI) and a high mitotic index. Thus, HER2 status is associated with the status of other biological parameters, which may explain the independent prognostic value of HER2 status and the lack of such value for other parameters. Indeed, many pathological and biological variables are commonly coexpressed in breast carcinomas and multiple correspondence analysis has identified features that are commonly clustered in HER2-positive tumors. Those variables frequently associated with HER2 overexpression are high histologic grade, necrosis, lymphocyte infiltration, high mitotic index, p53 mutation and lack of hormone receptor and bcl-2 expression [Ménard et al. 1999]. HER2 overexpression was not associated with tumor size, lymph node status, tumor vascularity, adhesion receptor expression, alteration in FHIT (fragile histidine triad), or the overexpression of phosphatases.

Table 1. Prognostic impact of HER2 in terms of mortality at 10 years according to nodal status and lymphoid infiltration

Tumor status	% mortality at 10 years		Increase in mortality in HER2+ patients compared to HER2– patients, %
	HER2+ patients	HER2– patients	
N+	67	45	49
N–	28	23	22
N–/LI–	32	22	45
N–/LI+	19	26	-27

N+ = Node positive; N– = node negative; LI– = no lymphoid infiltrate; LI+ = lymphoid infiltrate.

HER2 Status and Lymphoid Infiltration

Rilke and coworkers [1991] have examined the association of LI with HER2 positivity in breast cancer patients. This analysis revealed that in HER2-positive, node-positive patients, prognosis was similar whether or not LI was present. However, in node-negative patients, the impact of LI is related to HER2 status (table 1). Specifically, patients with LI who are HER2 positive have a better prognosis than those who are HER2 negative (27% decreased probability of death at 10 years), whereas HER2-positive patients without LI have a significantly worse prognosis than HER2-negative patients. It is plausible that these results reflect the immunogenic potential of

Table 2. Phenotypic features of tumor subsets identified in a retrospective study of primary breast cancer samples

Phenotype A	Phenotype B
Low grade	High grade
Low mitotic index	High mitotic index
No necrosis	Necrosis
No lymphoid infiltrate	Lymphoid infiltrate
p53–	p53+
HER2–	HER2+
PgR+	PgR–
Bcl-2+	Bcl-2–

PgR = Progesterone receptor.

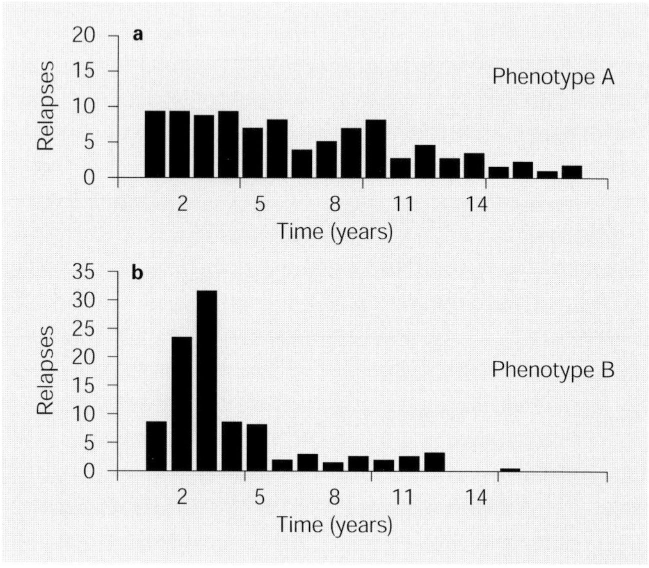

Fig. 2. Incidence of relapse in breast cancer patients with (**a**) phenotype A or (**b**) phenotype B tumors.

HER2. These data suggest that the HER2 protein may be the target of immune surveillance, which balances the invasive phenotype characteristic of HER2-overexpressing tumors. This raises the possibility that increasing the immunogenic potential of HER2 may result in an active immunotherapy.

Two Breast Cancer Subsets with Divergent Clinical Behaviour

Many pathologic and biologic variables are commonly associated and coexpressed in breast cancer subtypes [Ménard et al. 1999]. Multiple correspondence analysis has revealed that HER2 protein overexpression clusters with seven other pathologic variables including histologic grade, necrosis, LI, mitotic index, PgR and bcl2 expression [Ménard et al. 1999]. Two distinct breast cancer phenotypes, designated phenotypes A and B, can be distinguished using an index calculated based on the expression of HER2 and associated pathologic and biologic variables (table 2). Phenotype A is characterized by tumors with the biologic features of normal breast epithelial cells, i.e. these tumors do not overexpress HER2 and show a relatively high degree of differentiation, slow proliferation, low levels of necrosis and LI, and no genetic alterations. In contrast, phenotype B tumors are quite distinct from normal tissue. They overexpress HER2, are poorly differentiated, and show evidence of more rapid proliferation, more frequent genetic alterations and a host immune reaction.

Marked differences in disease outcome are evident when patients are grouped according to these tumor phenotypes. Patients in the high-risk, HER2-positive group tend to be younger and are significantly more likely to suffer relapse in the first 2–3 years following surgery, compared with the HER2-negative group who show a low rate of relapse in the year following surgery that remains constant over time (fig. 2). Overall survival of patients with HER2-positive, phenotype B tumors was reduced compared with patients with HER2-negative phenotype A tumors.

Preliminary data suggest that these tumor phenotypes may also predict for response to therapy. Patients treated prior to surgery with doxorubicin were classified according to clinical response and tumor phenotype (table 2). The majority of patients experiencing complete responses had tumors expressing the HER2-positive phenotype B (63%), whereas the incidence of phenotype B tumors was lower (34%) in patients who did not respond to therapy. These findings are consistent with independent observations that chemotherapy reduces the rate of early relapse of breast carcinomas and that HER2-positive tumors respond better to chemotherapy [Muss et al. 1994; Paik et al. 1998; Ravdin et al. 1998].

HER2 and Progression of Early Breast Cancer Lesions to Invasive Carcinomas

HER2 gene amplification/overexpression is an early event in the development of breast cancer and may be a marker for predicting clinical course in patients with early disease [Allred et al. 1992b; Barnes et al. 1992; Liu et al. 1992; Maguire et al. 1992]. Histologic studies have identified two precursor lesions of infiltrating ductal carcinomas (IDC). The first type occurs in older patients and progresses slowly on account of its estrogen dependency. However, it is more aggressive long term. The other type of IDC is found in younger patients and is HER2 positive. Atypical ductal hyperplasia (ADH) is a monoclonal lesion that is considered to be a precursor to IDC. DCIS appears as a focus of proliferating, presumably malignant epithelial cells that is confined to the mammary ducts and lobules and shows no evidence of invasion through the basement membrane into the surrounding stroma.

A major issue in the clinical management of DCIS is the risk of progression to invasive carcinoma. A positive HER2 status has been associated with the comedo subtype of DCIS, which has a more malignant phenotype and is more frequently associated with areas of micro-invasion [Barnes et al. 1992; van de Vijver et al. 1988]. HER2 amplification/overexpression has not been detected in ADH, whereas it is expressed in 70% of DCIS lesions and 30% of invasive ductal carcinoma lesions. These statistics present an interesting paradox. They suggest that the HER2-positive phenotype develops during the progression from ADH to DCIS, but may be frequently lost during progression to IDC, perhaps as a result of HER2-directed immune response. An alternative hypothesis is that HER2-negative IDCs do not derive from DCIS, but develop from ADH via an alternative pathway. This second hypothesis is supported by evidence that HER2 status is similar in both the in situ and invasive components of a single tumor (Allred et al. 1992b; Barnes et al. 1992; Liu et al. 1992]. The pathobiologic features of DCIS are similar to the HER2-positive subset of breast carcinoma, indicating that they may be derived from this precursor lesion (table 3). The HER2-negative subset of invasive carcinomas appear to derive from ADH, as they also share many characteristics. Thus, there are two precursors that could arise due to different mechanisms of transformation and produce two subsets of IDC.

Table 3. Pathobiological characteristics of ADH and DCIS

ADH	DCIS
Low grade	High grade
Low mitotic index	High mitotic index
No lymphoid infiltration	Lymphoid infiltration
No necrosis	Necrosis
p53–	p53+
HER2–	HER2+

Conclusions

Studies on the relationship between HER2 and the patholobiologic features of breast cancer have provided insight into the factors influencing the prognosis and progression of breast carcinoma. In node-negative patients, the prognostic value of HER2 remains controversial. A large, retrospective analysis confirmed that HER2 independently predicts poor prognosis in node-positive breast cancer patients. Lymphoid infiltration is frequently present in HER2-positive tumors and strongly influences the prognostic impact of HER2. In the absence of lymphoid infiltration, HER2 overexpression is clearly indicative of a poor prognosis in both node-positive and node-negative patients. In contrast, in the presence of lymphoid cells at the tumor site, HER2 overexpression is associated with an improved prognosis. This suggests that the aggressive phenotype characteristic of HER2-positive breast carcinomas may be balanced by immune surveillance against early stage, HER2-positive tumors.

Multiple correspondence analysis showed that HER2 amplification/overexpression is strongly associated with a range of prognostic features in breast cancers and identifies a subset of breast carcinomas quite divergent from the HER2-negative tumor phenotype. Patients with high-risk, HER2-positive tumors are younger, significantly more likely to suffer early relapse, and have reduced overall survival (phenotype B) compared with patients with HER2-negative phenotype A tumors. The characteristics of the HER2-positive tumors are also found in DCIS, suggesting that HER2-positive invasive carcinomas derive specifically from this precursor lesion.

Due to its prognostic significance, HER2 determination should be incorporated into the routine assessment of breast carcinoma. Evaluation of HER2 status in combination with other prognostic markers enhances the accuracy and power of the predictive prognosis and should help to more clearly define the most appropriate treatment for the individual patient.

References

Allred DC, Clark GM, Molina R, Tandon AK, Schnitt SJ, Gilchrist KW, Osborne CK, Tormey DC, McGuire WL: Overexpression of HER2/*neu* and its relationship with other prognostic factors changed during progression of in situ to invasive breast cancer. Hum Pathol 1992a;23:974–979.

Allred DC, Clark GM, Tandon AK, Molina R, Tormey DC, Osborne CK, Gilchrist KW, Mansour EG, Abeloff M, Eudey L, et al: HER-2/neu in node-negative breast cancer: prognostic significance of overexpression influenced by the presence of in situ carcinoma. J Clin Oncol 1992b;10:599–605.

Barnes DM, Bartkova J, Camplejohn RS, Gullick WJ, Smith PJ, Millis RR: Overexpression of c-erbB-2 oncoprotein: why does this occur more frequently in ductal carcinoma in situ than in invasive mammary carcinoma and is this of prognostic significance? Eur J Cancer 1992;28: 644–648.

Clark GM, McGuire WL: Prognostic factors in primary breast cancer. Breast Cancer Res Treat 1983;3:S69–S72.

Coussens L, Yang-Feng TL, Liao Y-C, Chen E, Gray A, McGrath J, Seeburg PH, Libermann TA, Schlessinger J, Francke U, et al: Tyrosine kinase receptor with extensive homology to EGF receptor shares chromosomal location with *neu* oncogene. Science 1985;230:1132–1139.

Di Fiore PP, Pierce JH, Fleming TP, Hazan R, Ullrich A, King CR, Schlessinger J, Aaronson SA: Overexpression of the human EGF receptor confers an EGF-dependent transformed phenotype to NIH3T3 cells. Cell 1987;51:1063–1070.

DiAugustine R, Richards RG: EGF-related peptides and their receptors in mammary gland development. J Mammary Gland Biol Neoplasia 1997;2:109–118.

Graus-Porta D, Beerli RR, Daly JM, Hynes NE: ErbB-2, the preferred heterodimerization partner of all ErbB receptors, is a mediator of lateral signalling. EMBO J 1997;16:1647–1655.

Hudziak RM, Schlessinger J, Ullrich A: Increased expression of the putative growth factor receptor $p185^{HER2}$ causes transformation and tumorigenesis of NIH3T3 cells. Proc Natl Acad Sci USA 1987;84:7159–7163.

Hynes NE, Stern DF: The biology of *erbB-2/neu/HER-2* and its role in cancer. Biochim Biophys Acta 1994;1198:165–184.

Liu E, Thor A, He M, Barcos M, Ljung BM, Benz CC: The HER2 (c-*erb*B-2) oncogene is frequently amplified in in situ carcinomas of the breast. Oncogene 1992;7:1027–1032.

Maguire HC, Hellman ME, Greene MI, Yeh I: Expression of c-*erb*B-2 in in situ and in adjacent invasive ductal adenocarcinomas of the female breast. Pathobiology 1992;60:117–121.

Ménard S, Casalini P, Tomasic G, Pilotti S, Cascinelli N, Buffalino RF, Longhi C, Rilke F, Colnaghi MI: Pathobiologic identification of two distinct breast carcinomas with diverging clinical behaviours. Breast Cancer Res Treat 1999; 55:169–177.

Muss H, Thor AD, Berry DA, Kute T, Liu ET, Koerner F, Cirrincione CT, Budman DR, Wood WC, Barcos M, et al: c-*erb*B-2 expression and response to adjuvant therapy in women with node-positive early breast cancer. N Engl J Med 1994;330:1260–1266.

Normanno E, Ciardiello F: EGF-related peptides in the pathophysiology of the mammary gland. J Mammary Gland Biol Neoplasia 1997;2:143–152.

Paik S, Bryant J, Park C, Fisher B, Tan-Chiu E,Hyams D, Fisher ER, Lipmann ME, Wickerham DL, Wolmark N: erbB-2 and response to doxorubicin in patients with axillary lymph node-positive, hormone receptor-negative breast cancer. J Natl Cancer Inst 1998;90: 1361–1370.

Ravdin PM, Green S, Albain KS, Boucher V, Ingle J, Pritchard K, Shepard L, Davidson N, Hayes DF, Clark GM, Martino S, Osborne CK, Allred DC: Initial report of the SWOG biological correlative study of C-erbB-2 expression as a predictor of outcome in a trial comparing adjuvant CAF T with tamoxifen (T) alone. Proc Am Soc Clin Oncol 1998;17:97A.

Rilke F, Colnaghi MI, Cascinelli N, Andreola S, Baldini MT, Bufalino R, Della Porta G, Menard S, Pierotti MA, Testori A: Prognostic significance of HER-2/*neu* expression in breast cancer and its relationship to other prognostic factors. Int J Cancer 1991;49:44–49.

Ross JS, Fletcher JA: The HER-2/neu oncogene in breast cancer: prognostic factor, predictive factor, and target for therapy. Stem Cells 1998;16: 413–428.

Slamon DJ, Clark GM, Wong SG, Levin WJ, Ullrich A, McGuire WL: Human breast cancer: correlation of relapse and survival with amplification of the HER-2/*neu* oncogene. Science 1987;235:177–182.

Slamon DJ, Godolphin W, Jones LA, Holt LA, Wong SG, Keith DE, Levin WJ, Stuart SG, Udove J, Ullrich A, et al: Studies of the HER-2/*neu* proto-oncogene in human breast and ovarian cancer. Science 1989;244:707–712.

Thorpe SM: Estrogen and progesterone receptor determinations in breast cancer. Technology, biology and clinical significance. Acta Oncol 1988;27:1–19.

van de Viyver MJ, Peterse JL, Mooi WJ, Wisman P, Lomans J, Dalesio O, Nusse R: Neu-protein overexpression in breast cancer. Association of the comedo-type ductal carcinoma and limited prognostic value in stage II breast cancer. N Engl J Med 1988;319:1239–1245.

Yarden Y: Biology of HER2 and its importance in breast cancer. Oncology 2001;61(suppl 2):1–13.

Oncology

Oncology 2001;61(suppl 2):73–82

The Predictive Value of HER2 in Breast Cancer

Martine Piccart Caroline Lohrisch Angelo Di Leo Denis Larsimont

Institut Jules Bordet, Brussels, Belgium

Key Words
Breast cancer · Predictive · HER2 · Herceptin® · Endocrine therapy · Chemotherapy · CMF · Adjuvant therapy · Algorithm

Abstract
Measurement of molecular markers predictive of response to therapy should enable more selective and effective utilization of anticancer agents. The predictive value of HER2 remains a complex and inconclusive subject. In metastatic breast cancer, HER2-positive, ER-positive patients can show responses to endocrine treatment, but experience shorter time to progression and survival than HER2-negative patients. In the adjuvant setting, weak, retrospective evidence suggests that tamoxifen is potentially harmful in HER2-positive patients and that there is no benefit from prolonged tamoxifen therapy. It has not yet been demonstrated conclusively that HER2 positivity increases resistance to adjuvant cyclophosphamide, methotrexate, 5-FU (CMF), but there are indications that HER2-positive patients benefit more from adequately dosed anthracyclines than from CMF. The greatest value of HER2 as a predictive marker lies in the prediction of response to therapies that target HER2, such as Herceptin®. Patients with strongly HER2-positive breast cancer derive significant clinical benefit from single-agent and combined Herceptin therapy. HER2 testing has become an integral part of the optimal management of the breast cancer patient. Best current practice in adjuvant breast cancer therapy based on the current knowledge of the potential predictive power of HER2 constitutes not denying tamoxifen to HER2-positive, ER-positive patients or CMF to HER2-positive patients. Outside of clinical trials, adequately dosed anthracycline-based chemotherapy is the current preferred adjuvant treatment option for HER2-positive patients.

Introduction

While significant developments such as the introduction of new chemotherapeutic agents and treatment regimens have led to improvements in breast cancer care in recent decades [Hortobagyi 2000], the Surveillance, Epidemiology and End Results database of the National Cancer Institute indicates that 45–50% of all patients diagnosed with breast cancer will develop refractory or resistant disease [Chu et al. 1999; Ries et al. 1999]. This worrying statistic highlights not only the continuing need for new and modified anticancer therapies and regimens, but also the importance of accurately assessing patient risk on presentation and choosing systemic therapy that is optimal for individual patients.

KARGER
Fax + 41 61 306 12 34
E-Mail karger@karger.ch
www.karger.com

0030–2414/01/0616–0073$17.50/0

Accessible online at:
www.karger.com/journals/ocl

M. Piccart, MD
Institut Jules Bordet
1 Rue Heger-Bordet
B–1000 Brussels (Belgium)
Tel. +32 2 541 3111, Fax +32 2 538 0858, E-Mail Mpiccart@ulb.ac.be

In the assessment of breast cancer patients, axillary node status, tumor size, tumor grade, and hormone receptor status are well-established prognostic factors [Ellegde et al. 1992]. Recently, however, a number of probes have been developed to detect molecular abnormalities in cancerous cells. These molecular markers can provide prognostic and/or predictive information. The search for novel markers with prognostic and/or predictive value also has critical importance in the development of effective anticancer treatments. For example, the introduction of novel biological agents such as the humanized anti-HER2 monoclonal antibody, Herceptin®, has marked the beginning of targeted therapy in hormone-resistant breast cancer care [Brenner and Adams 1999].

The investigation of the potential of molecular markers such as p53 and human epidermal growth factor receptor-2 (HER2) to predict sensitivity or resistance to various systemic treatments for breast cancer continues to be an active area of research. Given their potential clinical utility, several groups have examined the relationship between tumor markers and response to various therapies and have categorized them on the strength of published evidence regarding their clinical usefulness [Bast et al. 2001; Fitzgibbons et al. 2000; Henson et al. 1995; Hayes et al. 1996, 1998; McGuire 1991; Piccart et al. 1999]. However, very few have actually been validated clinically and technically for routine clinical assessment in breast cancer. At present, only estrogen receptor (ER) and progesterone receptor status are fully accepted as having prognostic and predictive value. Both of these receptors predict for a response to hormonal therapy [Hayes et al. 1996].

Clinical Validation of HER2

HER2 is amplified/overexpressed in 20–30% of breast cancer patients [Slamon et al. 1987, 1989]. HER2 overexpression is the result of gene amplification and/or enhanced transcription, whereas gene amplification results from an increased number of gene copies per chromosome or aneuploidy [Hynes and Stern 1994; Pauletti et al. 1996; Vona et al. 1999]. In vitro studies in breast cancer cells indicate that HER2 amplification is present in the vast majority (92%) of breast cancers with HER2 overexpression [Pauletti et al. 1996]. Current evidence supports a clear association between HER2 amplification/overexpression and reduced overall and disease-free survival, especially in patients with node-positive disease [Hynes 1993; Hynes and Stern 1994; Slamon et al. 1987, 1989; for a review, see Ross and Fletcher 1998]. Interestingly, it appears that only tumors displaying HER2 amplification show a correlation with poor prognosis [Borg et al. 1990; Farabegoli et al. 1999].

While it has generally been accepted that HER2 amplification/overexpression is correlated with a poor prognosis in breast cancer, it has not yet been possible to draw definite conclusions with regard to the influence of HER2 positivity on the response to endocrine or chemotherapy [Piccart et al. 2000]. Interpretation of the data currently available has been confounded by many factors, including retrospective studies done on subsets of clinical trial populations, small patient numbers, poorly reported study conditions and the use of different HER2 testing approaches. The potential impact of HER2 status on the planning of individualized treatment underscores the need to refine and standardize HER2 testing in order to minimize false-negative results [for a review, see Hanna 2001]. Clearly, well-standardized assay systems and quality-control programs to assess whether individual laboratories can perform HER2 testing and scoring accurately and reproducibly are required.

The College of American Pathologists has assigned a category II ranking to HER2, meaning that additional evidence is required to support its clinical value [Fitzgibbons et al. 2000]. However, the recent update of the American Society of Clinical Oncology Recommendations for the use of tumor markers in breast cancer has reached the conclusion that the HER2 status of all primary breast cancers should be determined at diagnosis or on recurrence and that HER2 overexpression and amplification can be used to identify patients for Herceptin therapy [Bast et al. 2001]. Thus, there is a growing consensus that HER2 is approaching a clinically validated status as a prognostic factor as well as a predictive factor for response to some systemic therapies. This acknowledgement of the clinical relevance of HER2 means that HER2 testing is already part of the routine assessment for breast cancer patients.

Recent research has begun to answer some of the open questions regarding HER2 and response to therapy [for a review, see Dowsett et al. 2000; Piccart et al. 2000; Ross and Fletcher 1998]. Large, randomized clinical trials [Cobleigh et al. 1999; Norton et al. 1999; Slamon et al. 1998] have shown that metastatic breast cancer patients with HER2-positive tumors obtain meaningful clinical benefits from the humanized monoclonal anti-HER2 antibody, Herceptin. Furthermore, HER2 positivity also appears to predict for resistance to treatment with cyclophosphamide, methotrexate and 5-FU (CMF) [Allred et al. 1992a; Giai et al. 1994; Gusterson et al. 1992; Stål et al.

Table 1. Meta-analysis of the interaction between HER2 and response to endocrine therapy in patients with metastatic breast cancer [De Laurentiis et al. 2000]

Study	Endocrine agent	Odds ratio for disease progression, HER2+ vs. HER2– patients	95% CI
Archer et al. 1995	Tamoxifen	1.81	0.66–4.92
Berns et al. 1995	Tamoxifen	4.20	1.44–12.28
Elledge et al. 1998	Tamoxifen	1.44	0.74–2.82
Houston et al. 1999	Tamoxifen	2.04	1.17–3.56
Leitzel et al. 1995	Megestrol acetate or fadrozole	2.65	1.34–5.26
Wright et al. 1992	Ovarian ablation or tamoxifen	7.72	0.93–63.78
Yamauchi et al. 1997	Droloxifene	6.75	2.44–18.64
Overall (n = 1,110)		2.46	1.81–3.34

1995] and tamoxifen [Bianco et al. 2000]. In particular, data presented at the American Society of Clinical Oncology 2000 meeting have shed some light on the predictive role of HER2. This paper provides an overview of the current knowledge pertaining to HER2 and the response to endocrine therapy, chemotherapy and Herceptin therapy, and reviews what constitutes best practice in adjuvant breast cancer therapy based on this understanding.

Predictive Value of HER2 for Endocrine Therapy

The hypothesis that HER2 overexpression leads to resistance to endocrine therapy has been strongly supported by in vitro studies which have indicated that conversion of MCF-7 cells to a HER2-overexpressing phenotype, by transfection of HER2 cDNA, led to estrogen-independent and tamoxifen-insensitive growth [Benz et al. 1992]. In breast cancer patients, several, but not all, clinical trials have also demonstrated an association between HER2 positivity and a significantly reduced response to tamoxifen and other endocrine therapies [Hamilton and Piccart 2000].

Advanced Breast Cancer

Retrospective analysis of the largest trials of endocrine therapy for advanced breast cancer has suggested that response rates to endocrine therapy were decreased in HER2-positive patients, in comparison with HER2-negative patients, in two out of the four largest trials [Leitzel et al. 1995; Houston et al. 1999] while the other two trials refuted this observation [Archer et al. 1995; Elledge et al. 1998]. A meta-analysis has recently been carried out on published data from seven studies on the interaction between HER2 and the response to endocrine therapy in 1,110 patients with metastatic breast cancer, most of whom received tamoxifen [De Laurentiis et al. 2000]. The studies included in this meta-analysis were identified by an extensive search of Medline and Embase for studies in metastatic breast cancer patients treated with endocrine therapy that involved assessment of response rates according to HER2 status. For each study, the odds of disease progression were taken as an indicator of the tumor resistance to the treatment and the odds ratio for HER2-positive over HER2-negative patients with 95% confidence interval (95% CI) was calculated as an estimate of the predictive effect of HER2. The study indicated that, overall, HER2-positive patients had a 2.46 times higher risk of disease progression on endocrine therapy than HER2-negative patients (table 1) [De Laurentiis et al. 2000]. However, it remains unclear whether this apparent higher risk represented true resistance to endocrine therapy or an overall poorer prognosis in HER2-positive patients in comparison with HER2-negative patients.

Another recent study measured serum HER2 levels in pretreatment sera from 566 metastatic breast cancer patients enrolled in two randomized, second-line endocrine therapy trials [Lipton et al. 2000]. 168/566 patients (30%) had elevated serum HER2 levels and the response rate (complete response + partial response + stable disease) was significantly less in the HER2-elevated patients (41/168; 24%) in comparison with patients with normal serum HER2 (176/398; 44%; $p < 0.0001$). Among the responding patients, the duration of response was also significantly shorter for patients with elevated HER2 and, in all patients, time to progression and overall survival were also significantly shorter for patients with elevated serum HER2 versus patients with normal levels. A multivariate analysis for response rate, time to progression and overall survival was performed which included serum HER2, age, race, disease-free interval, performance status, visceral versus non-visceral metastasis and ER/PR status as variables. After adjustment for the other variables, elevated serum HER2 remained an independent predictor of the outcome of endocrine therapy.

Adjuvant Therapy for Early Breast Cancer

New insights into the predictive value of HER2 have also recently come to light in the setting of adjuvant endocrine therapy for early breast cancer. The 20-year follow-up data from the Naples GUN trial have recently been reported [Bianco et al. 2000]. In this prospective, randomized study conducted between 1978 and 1983, 433 patients were assigned to treatment with tamoxifen for two years or no tamoxifen with nine cycles of CMF. Tumor blocks could only be retrieved for 245 patients, and only 63 were HER2-positive, but there was a clear interaction between HER2 positivity and outcome on adjuvant tamoxifen. Mean (95% CI) hazard ratios for death in HER2-positive and HER2-negative patients were 1.09 (0.63–1.87) and 0.59 (0.40–0.87), respectively ($p = 0.04$). Thus, the relative risk of death was clearly reduced with tamoxifen treatment in HER2-negative women but not in HER2-positive women [Bianco et al. 2000].

In addition, a Swedish prospective randomized trial of tamoxifen for two years and five years, in which tumor blocks were retrieved and tested for HER2 in 519/1,662 patients, has also reported that HER2-negative patients benefited from prolonged tamoxifen treatment while HER2-positive patients did not [Nordenskjold et al. 2000].

In conclusion, in relation to endocrine therapy for breast cancer, preclinical studies indicate there is a clear biological basis for a relationship between HER2 overexpression and resistance to endocrine treatment. In metastatic breast cancer, retrospective clinical studies suggest that although HER2-positive, ER-positive patients can show objective responses to endocrine treatment, they experience shorter time to progression and shorter survival than their HER2-negative counterparts. In the adjuvant setting there is weak, retrospective evidence to suggest that tamoxifen is potentially ineffective in HER2-positive patients and that there is no benefit from prolonged (five years) tamoxifen therapy. Further studies are being planned, which aim to clarify the complex issue of the relationship between HER2 overexpression and possible resistance to endocrine therapy. For example, the European Organisation for Research and Treatment of Cancer (EORTC) is planning a trial in which HER2-positive patients, who are progressing while receiving adjuvant tamoxifen, or on tamoxifen for advanced breast cancer, will receive concomitant therapy with Herceptin in order to see whether Herceptin can reverse resistance to tamoxifen. In addition, a trial of the oral aromatase inhibitor, anastrozole, given with or without Herceptin, is also about to be started in HER2-positive, ER-positive patients with metastatic breast cancer. However, at the present time, in terms of daily patient management, there is still insufficient evidence to deny endocrine therapy to HER2-positive, ER-positive breast cancer patients in the advanced or adjuvant settings although such patients do require careful follow-up.

Predictive Value of HER2 for Chemotherapy

The evidence to support HER2 as a marker for response to chemotherapy is weaker than that for endocrine therapy and has been derived mainly from the adjuvant setting because data in metastatic disease are scarce [Hamilton and Piccart 2000; Piccart et al. 2000] Three assumptions about the predictive value of HER2 in relation to chemotherapy will be discussed here, which are currently a matter for debate amongst oncologists. These include: the potential for HER2 positivity to predict for resistance to CMF; that HER2 positivity predicts for sensitivity to 'adequately dosed' anthracycline-based chemotherapy; and finally, that HER2-positive patients benefit more from anthracycline- than CMF-based regimens.

HER2 and Resistance to CMF

In the adjuvant chemotherapy setting, retrospective analyses of three trials have suggested that adjuvant CMF provided benefit in HER2-positive patients [Ménard et al. 1999; Allred et al. 1992b; Miles et al. 1999] and one trial has suggested there was no significant benefit [Gusterson et al. 1992] (table 2). Although the study reported by Ménard et al. [1999] was relatively small-scale in terms of the number of HER2-positive patients included, it was valuable in that it involved a 20-year follow-up, 87% of tumor blocks were retrieved, and CMF (without prednisone) was compared with no treatment. Furthermore, the decreased hazard ratios indicated that HER2-positive patients did gain some benefit from CMF therapy (table 2). On the contrary, the study that was reported by Gusterson et al. [1992] suggested that it was the HER2-negative patients who benefited from prolonged CMF therapy. However, in this study only 61% of tumor blocks were

Table 2. HER2 and CMF-based chemotherapy

Author/group (follow-up)	Population/ percentage tested for HER2 HER2 assay	Treatment arms	n total/ HER2+	Disease-free survival			
				HER2+		HER2–	
Gusterson et al. 1992 (6 years)	Node + 61 IHC (MAb)	CMFP 1 cycle perioperative CMFP 6 post- + 1 perioperative	255/55 491/85	29% 38%	ns	36% 52%	0.0001
Allred et al. 1992b (5 years)	Node – 16 IHC (poly Ab)	Nil (low risk[a]) Nil CMFP	307/40 146/35 160/40	~ 76% ~ 70% ~ 78%	NS	~ 82% ~ 60% ~ 80%	0.0003
Ménard et al. 1999 (20 years)	Node + 87 IHC (?)	Nil CMF	155/25 180/29	HR[b] = 0.48		HR[b] = 0.64	
Miles et al. 1999 (5 years)	Node + ? IHC	Nil CMF	147/83 130/	35% 65%	0.007	65% 85%	<0.01

IHC = immunohistochemistry.
[a] Low-risk patients had ER-positive tumors <3 cm.
[b] Hazard ratio (CMF versus no CMF).
[c] 83 tumors were HER2 positive. Numbers of HER2+ and HER2– women were similar in both treatment groups.

retrieved and, as only 140/746 patients were HER2-positive, the statistical power of the study to compare the outcomes of the HER2-positive patients in the two treatment arms was clearly much less than the statistical power to compare the outcomes in the HER2-negative patients (table 2).

The findings of the study by Allred et al. (1992b) were rather less clear-cut in that patients were stratified into low- and high-risk groups according to tumor size and estrogen-receptor (ER) status. High-risk patients (ER-negative or large [≥ 3 cm] ER-positive tumors) were randomized either to observation only or treatment with CMF prednisone. In addition, patients were followed-up for 5 years and only 16% of tumor blocks were retrieved. In the HER2-negative subgroup, CMF plus prednisone-treated patients in the high-risk category benefited in that their disease-free survival was similar to untreated patients in the low-risk (ER-positive tumors <3cm) category (table 2). In contrast, in the HER2-positive subgroup, none of the comparisons was statistically significant, possibly because of the low patient number. However, the CMF plus prednisone-treated patients in the high-risk category appeared to have disease-free survival similar to untreated patients in the low-risk category (table 2).

HER2 and Sensitivity to Anthracyclines

The evidence that HER2 positivity is predictive for sensitivity to anthracycline-based chemotherapy appears to be more straightforward. A study reported by Paik et al. [1998], which involved 13.5 years mean follow-up, indicated that disease-free survival was significantly longer in node-positive, HER2-positive breast cancer patients treated with L-phenylalanine mustard, 5-fluorouracil and doxorubicin (PAF) than in those treated with L-phenylalanine mustard, 5-fluorouracil (PF). Similarly, a recent Belgian study that compared epirubicin plus cyclophosphamide (EC) with CMF in node-positive breast cancer patients, followed for four years, indicated that event-free survival was better in HER2-positive patients treated with high-dose EC than CMF [Di Leo et al. 1999]. Furthermore, it has been suggested that there was an improvement in disease-free survival in post-menopausal, HER2-positive patients who were treated with the combination of adjuvant anthracycline chemotherapy (cyclophosphamide, doxorubicin, fluorouracil [CAF]) plus tamoxifen in comparison with tamoxifen alone [Ravdin et al. 1998].

HER2 and Anthracycline Dose-Response

In addition, three further studies have suggested that HER2-positive tumors are particularly sensitive to anthracycline dose intensity [Clahsen et al. 1998; Thor et al. 1998; Petit et al. 2000] (table 3). These studies indicated that HER2-positive patients do not seem to benefit from only one cycle of perioperative CAF chemotherapy [Clahsen et al. 1998] or low-dose CAF [Thor et al. 1998] but do benefit from standard/high-dose CAF and high-dose neo-adjuvant FEC chemotherapy [Petit et al. 2000]. Moreover, the dose-response effect for anthracyclines was much less evident in the HER2-negative patient population.

In summary, to date, tumor blocks from more than 6,000 breast cancer patients enrolled in prospective trials of adjuvant chemotherapy have been retrieved and analysed for HER2 status. Of these, 1,369 women were declared to be HER2 positive. The results from this population have not yet provided a definitive answer as to whether HER2 positivity increases resistance to CMF, but they do suggest that such patients benefit more from anthracyclines than CMF, and that they require treatment with adequate doses of anthracyclines. It is now clear that prospective clinical trials are needed to validate the hypothesis that HER2-positive patients benefit more from anthracycline-based chemotherapy than CMF. The biological basis of the relationship between HER2 and anthracycline sensitivity may also be worthy of further investigation as it has been suggested that amplification of topoisomerase II, the target enzyme for anthracyclines, occurs in approximately 40% of HER2-overexpressing tumors [Jarvinen et al. 2000].

Predictive Value of HER2 for Herceptin Therapy

The greatest value of HER2 as a predictive marker in patients with breast cancer obviously lies in the prediction of response to therapies that target the HER2 receptor protein, such as the humanized monoclonal antibody, Herceptin. Prior knowledge of HER2 status is an absolute requirement for Herceptin therapy and testing for HER2 status should now be part of the routine clinical assessment for breast cancer patients [Bast et al. 2001].

The level of benefit obtained from Herceptin therapy correlates with the level of HER2 overexpression as determined by immunohistochemistry (IHC) or presence or absence of HER2 gene amplification, as determined by fluorescence in situ hybridisation (FISH). In the pivotal phase II trial of single-agent Herceptin as second/third-line therapy for metastatic disease, Cobleigh et al. [1999] reported that higher levels of HER2 overexpression (i.e.

Table 3. HER2 and anthracycline-based chemotherapy dose-intensity

Author/group (follow-up)	Population/ percentage tested for HER2 HER2 assay	Treatment arms	n total/HER2+	Disease-free survival			
				HER2+		HER2–	
Clahsen et al. 1998 (4 years)	Node –, prem 65 IHC (MAb)	Nil CAF, perioperative	210/31 230/29	77% 90%	NS	78% 85%	0.05
Thor et al. 1998 (5 years)	Node + 63 IHC (MAb)	Low-dose CAF High + standard-dose CAF	322/88 670/184	50% 71%[a]	0.001	60% 65%[a]	0.058
Di Leo et al. 1999	Node + 62 IHC (MAb)	EC 60 High-dose EC 100	267/19 255/14	53% 81%	NA	67% 74%	NA
Petit et al. 2000	Large T2, T3 100 IHC (MAb)	FEC 50 FEC 100	79/24	0% 100% (RR)	0.07	75% 72% (RR)	NS

FEC = 5-FU, epirubicin, cyclophosphamide.

[a] High-dose CAF results only [Petit et al., 2000].

3+ versus 2+) predicted for a higher response rate (table 4). Significantly, retrospective analysis of the clinical efficacy of Herceptin in the pivotal phase II and III trials has revealed evidence that HER2 3+ patients obtain a higher level of clinical benefit from Herceptin therapy than the overall population comprising HER2 2+ and 3+ patients [Mass et al. 2000; Slamon et al. 2001; Roche, data on file] (table 4, 5). However, caution is required in the interpretation of such evidence derived from retrospective analyses. Interestingly, retesting of tissue samples from patients in the pivotal trials with FISH indicates that 24% of HER2 2+ patients are FISH positive. Furthermore, FISH-positive and IHC 3+ patients have similar outcomes on Herceptin therapy [Mass et al. 2000], indicating that the subset of HER2 2+ overexpressors who are also FISH positive may benefit from Herceptin. As in the phase III combination trial, a trial of single-agent Herceptin as first-line therapy for metastatic breast cancer has revealed a higher response rate in IHC 3+ patients relative to IHC 2+/3+ patients combined (35 versus 26%) [Vogel et al. 2000]. Interestingly, no responders were identified in the IHC 2+ patient population in this trial (table 4). Collectively, these trial data strongly support the concept that with HER2 testing by IHC, the level of HER2 overexpression is predictive of the response to Herceptin therapy.

Table 4. Efficacy of Herceptin monotherapy in HER2 3+ and HER2 2+ overexpressing breast cancer patients [Vogel et al. 2000[1]; Cobleigh et al. 1999[2]]

	Response rate, %	TTP months	OS months
Herceptin first line[1]			
HER2 3+ (n = 87)[1]	35	NA	NA
HER2 2+ (n = 27)[1]	0	NA	NA
Herceptin second line[2]			
IHC 3+ (n = 172)[2]	18	3.2	16.4
IHC 2+ (n = 50)[2]	6	1.9	8.8

OS = Overall survival; TTP = time to progression.

Adjuvant Breast Cancer Treatment Algorithm

As with ER status, it is likely that further studies will establish the importance of HER2 status as a predictor of response to therapy. Knowledge of HER2 status is essential in stratifying patients to anti-HER2 therapy regimens. Furthermore, HER2 receptor overexpression in invasive disease and ductal carcinoma in situ [van de Vijver et al. 1988] suggests that anti-HER2 therapy could potentially be of therapeutic benefit for the treatment of breast cancer at an early stage in the disease.

Based on the current understanding of the predictive power of HER2, it is possible to construct a treatment algorithm illustrating the best practice in adjuvant care of HER2-positive breast cancer patients (fig. 1). Herceptin is expected to have considerable therapeutic potential in the adjuvant setting and trials to investigate this are already at the planning stage [for a review, see Leyland-Jones and Smith 2001]. Therefore, the highest priority among clinicians should be to encourage HER2-positive patients to enter into randomized clinical trials to explore the benefit of Herceptin in adjuvant treatment of breast cancer. It is currently not recommended to deny tamoxifen to ER-positive patients, but patients with HER2-positive tumors receiving tamoxifen should be followed closely. Furthermore, based on the evidence discussed above, CMF should also not be denied to a HER2-positive patient. However, outside of the clinical-trial setting, the current preferred and most cautious adjuvant treatment option would be an adequately dosed anthracycline-based che-

Table 5. Efficacy of Herceptin (H) plus paclitaxel (P) in HER2 3+ and HER2 2+ overexpressing breast cancer patients (means and 95% CI) [Mass et al. 2000]

	HER2 3+		HER2 2+	
	H + P (n = 68)	P (n = 77)	H + P (n = 24)	P (n = 19)
Response rate, %	49 (36–61)	17 (9–27)	21 (7–42)	16 (3–40)
TTP, months	7.1 (6.2–12)	3 (2–4.4)	5.3 (3.4–6.6)	2.7 (2.0–5.3)
OS, months	25 (18.6–33.7)	18 (11.2–23.8)	17 (12.0–25.0)	20 (8.0–27.0)

OS = Overall survival; TTP = time to progression.

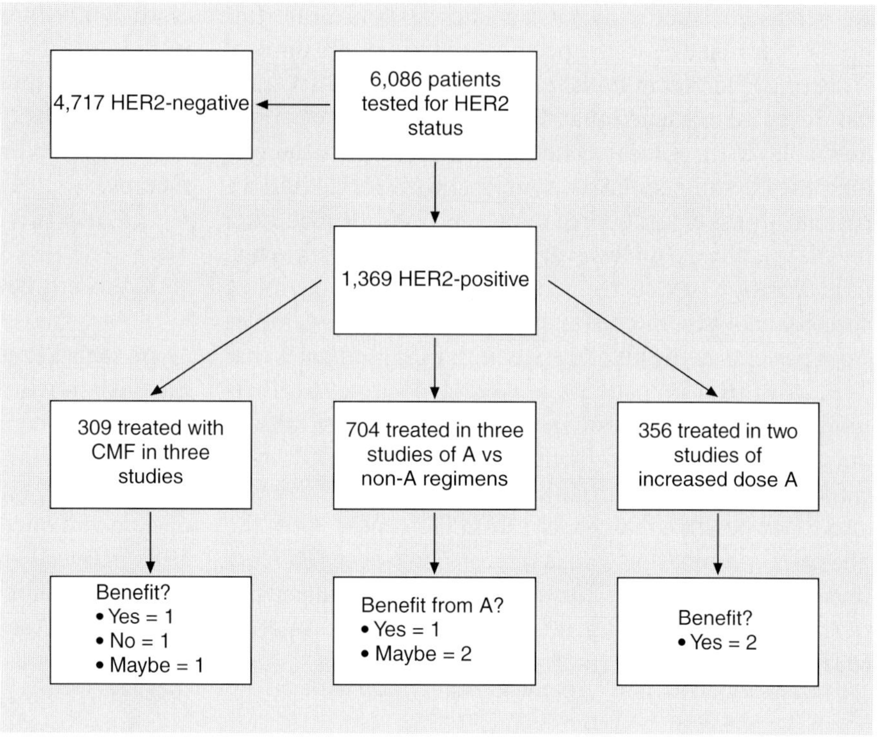

Fig. 1. Proposed guidelines for clinical practice in the adjuvant setting based on the use of HER2 as a predictive factor.

motherapy. The accumulation of new trial data will inevitably lead to the expansion and probable revision of the treatment algorithm presented here.

Conclusions

Measurement of molecular markers predictive of responsiveness to therapy allows for more individualized and effective anticancer therapy. There is general agreement that HER2 amplification/overexpression correlates with poor prognosis in breast cancer. However, it has not yet been possible to draw definite conclusions with regard to the impact of HER2 on response to endocrine or chemotherapy. The contradictions and ambiguities in the current data regarding the predictive utility of HER2 reflect, in particular, the high degree of inconsistency between, as well as insufficient reporting of HER2 testing methods, and the relatively small patient populations used in the numerous retrospective studies. The impact of HER2 status on individualizing treatment highlights the need to refine and standardize HER2 testing in order to minimize false-negative results.

Recently emerged data are beginning to address some of the open questions regarding the predictive value of HER2. Generally, HER2-positive status has been shown to predict for decreased response rates to hormonal therapy, especially tamoxifen. The relationship between HER2 status and chemotherapy appears to be weaker and less well defined. Several studies suggest that HER2 status predicts sensitivity to anthracycline-based treatment and resistance to CMF therapy, although other studies have found conflicting results. Large, quantitative, prospective studies are required to verify conclusively the association of HER2 with response to hormonal and chemotherapy.

The greatest and undisputable advantage of knowing HER2 status in patients with breast cancer lies in the prediction of response to therapies that target the HER2 receptor protein, such as Herceptin. Thus, HER2 testing has become an integral part of the optimal management of the breast cancer patient. The clinical data currently available have demonstrated that patients with strongly HER2-positive breast cancer derive a significant clinical benefit from single-agent Herceptin, as well as from therapies that combine Herceptin with other anticancer agents. Moreover, recent data derived from subset analyses of patients enrolled in the pivotal Herceptin trials strongly suggest that HER2 3+ overexpression predicts for greater benefit from Herceptin therapy. Subsequent testing with FISH may identify those IHC 2+ patients who are likely to benefit from Herceptin.

Applying the current knowledge of the predictive power of HER2 to patient management, it is possible to devise an algorithm of best current practice in adjuvant breast cancer therapy. Current evidence supports not denying tamoxifen to HER2-positive, ER-positive patients or CMF to HER2-positive patients. Outside of clinical trials, adequately dosed anthracycline-based chemotherapy is the preferred adjuvant treatment option at present. Given the potential therapeutic benefit of Herceptin in primary breast cancer, physicians should motivate patients to enter into adjuvant clinical trials of Herceptin.

References

Allred DC, Clark GM, Molina R, Tandon AK, Schnitt SJ, Gilchrist KW, Osborne CK, Tormey DC, McGuire WL: Overexpression of HER-2/neu and its relationship with other prognostic factors changed during progression of in-situ to invasive breast cancer. Hum Pathol 1992a;23:974–979.

Allred DC, Clark GM, Tandon AK, Molina R, Tormey DC, Osborne CK, Gilchrist KW, Mansour EG, Abeloff M, Eudey L, et al: HER-2/neu in node-negative breast cancer: prognostic significance of overexpression influenced by the presence of in situ carcinoma. J Clin Oncol 1992b; 10:599–605.

Archer SG, Eliopoulos A, Spandidos D, Barnes D, Ellis IO, Blamey RW, Nicholson RI, Robertson JF: Expression of ras p21, p53 and c-erbB-2 in advanced breast cancer and response to first-line hormonal therapy. Br J Cancer 1995;72: 1259–1266.

Bast RC, Jr, Ravdin P, Hayes DF, Bates S, Fritsche H, Jr, Jessup JM, Kemeny N, Locker GY, Mennel RG, Somerfield MR, for the American Society of Clinical Oncology Tumor Markers Expert Panel: 2000 Update of recommendations for the use of tumor markers in breast and colorectal cancer: Clinical Practice Guidelines of the American Society of Clinical Oncology. J Clin Oncol 2001;19:1865–1878.

Benz CC, Scott GK, Sarup JC, Johnson RM, Tripathy D, Coronado E, Shepard HM, Osborne CK: Estrogen-dependent, tamoxifen-resistant tumorigenic growth of MCF-7 cells transfected with HER2/*neu*. Breast Cancer Res Treat 1992;24:85–95.

Berns EM, Foekens JA, van Staveren IL, van Putten WL, de Koning HY, Portengen H, Klijn JG: Oncogene amplification and prognosis in breast cancer: relationship with systemic treatment. Gene 1995;159:11–18.

Bianco AR, De Laurentiis M, Carlomagno C, Gallo C, Panico L, De Placido S: HER2 overexpression predicts adjuvant tamoxifen (TAM) failure for early breast cancer (EBC): complete data at 20 yr of the Naples GUN randomized trial. Proc Am Soc Clin Oncol 2000;19:75A.

Borg A, Tandon AK, Sigurdsson H, Clark GM, Fernö M, Fuqua SAW, Killander D, McGuire WL: HER2/neu amplification predicts poor survival in node positive patients. Cancer Res 1990; 50:6701–6707.

Brenner TL, Adams VR: First MAb approved for the treatment of metastatic breast cancer. J Am Pharm Assoc 1999;39:236–238.

Chu KC, Tarone RE, Brawley OW: Breast cancer trends of black women compared with white women. Arch Fam Med 1999;8:521–528.

Clahsen PC, van de Velde CJH, Duval C, Pallud C, Mandard A-M, Delobelle-Deroide A, van den Broek L, Sahmoud TM, van de Vijver MJ: P53 protein accumulation and response to adjuvant chemotherapy in premenopausal women with node-negative early breast cancer. J Clin Oncol 1998;16:470–479.

Cobleigh MA, Vogel CL, Tripathy D, Robert NJ, Scholl S, Fehrenbacher L, Wolter JM, Paton V, Shak S, Lieberman G, Slamon DJ: Multinational study of the efficacy and safety of humanized anti-HER2 monoclonal antibody in women who have HER2-overexpressing metastatic breast cancer that has progressed after chemotherapy for metastatic disease. J Clin Oncol 1999;17:2639–2648.

De Laurentiis M, Arpino G, Massarelli E, Carlomagno C, Ciardiello F, Tortora G, Bianco AR, De Placido S: A metanalysis of the interaction between Her2 and the response to endocrine therapy (ET) in metastatic breast cancer (MBC). Proc Am Soc Clin Oncol 2000;19: 78A.

Di Leo A, Larsimont D, Beauduin M, Vindevoghel A, Michel J, Focan C, Tagnon A, Ries F, Gobert P, Closon-Dejardin MT, Dolci S, Bartholomeus S, Lobelle JP, Paesmans M, Piccart MJ: CMF or anthracycline-based adjuvant chemotherapy for node-positive (N+) breast cancer (BC) patients (PTS): 4 year results of a Belgian randomised clinical trial with predictive markers analysis. Proc Am Soc Clin Oncol 1999;18:69A.

Dowsett M, Cooke T, Ellis I, Gullick WJ, Gusterson B, Ballon E, Mallon E, Walker R: Assessment of HER2 status in breast cancer: why, when and how? Eur J Cancer 2000:36:160–176.

Elledge RM, McGuire WL and Osborne CK: Prognostic factors in breast cancer. Semin Oncol 1992;19:244–253.

Elledge RM, Green S, Ciocca D, Pugh R, Allred DC, Clark GM, Hill J, Ravdin P, O'Sullivan J, Martino S, Osborne CK: HER-2 expression and response to tamoxifen in estrogen receptor-positive breast cancer: a Southwest Oncology Group Study. Clin Cancer Res 1998;4:7–12.

Farabegoli F, Ceccarelli C, Santini D, Baldini N, Tafurelli M, Marrano D, Trere D, Derenzini M: c-erbB-2 overexpression in amplified and non-amplified breast carcinoma samples. Int J Cancer 1999;84:273–277.

Fitzgibbons PL, Page DL, Weaver D, Thor AD, Allred DC, Clark GM, Ruby SG, O'Malley F, Simpson JF, Connolly JL, Hayes DF, Edge SB, Lichter A, Schnitt SJ: Prognostic Factors in Breast Cancer. Arch Pathol Lab Med 2000;124: 966–978.

Giai M, Roagna R, Ponzone R, De Bortoli M, Dati C, Sismondi P: Prognostic and predictive relevance of c-erbB-2 and ras expression in node positive and negative breast cancer. Anticancer Res 1994;14:1441–1450.

Gusterson BA, Gelber RD, Goldhirsch A, Price KN, Save-Soderborgh J, Styles J, Rudenstam CM, Golouh R, Reed R, et al: Prognostic importance of c-erbB-2 expression in breast cancer. J Clin Oncol 1992;10:1049–1056.

Hamilton A, Piccart M: The contribution of molecular markers to the prediction of response in the treatment of breast cancer: a review of the literature on HER-2, p53 and BCL-2. Ann Oncol 2000;11:647–63.

Hanna W: Testing for HER2 status. Oncology 2001;61(suppl 2):22–30.

Hayes DF, Bast R, Desch CE: A tumor marker utility grading system (TMUGS): a framework to evaluate clinical utility of tumor markers. J Natl Cancer Inst 1996;88:1456–1466.

Hayes DF, Trock B, Harris AL: Assessing the clinical impact of prognostic factors: when is 'statistically significant' clinically useful? Breast Cancer Res Treat 1998;52:305–319.

Henson DE, Fielding P, Grignon DJ, Page DL, Hammond ME, Nash G, Pettigrew NM, Gorstein F, Hutter RV: College of American Pathologists Conference XXVI on clinical relevance of prognostic markers in solid tumors. Arch Pathol Lab Med 1995;19:1109–1112.

Hortobagyi, GN: Developments in chemotherapy of breast cancer. Cancer 2000;88(suppl 12): 3073–3079.

Houston SJ, Plunkett TA, Barnes DM, Smith P, Rubens RD, Miles DW: Overexpression of c-erbB2 is an independent marker of resistance to endocrine therapy in advanced breast cancer. Br J Cancer 1999;79:1220–1226.

Hynes NE, Stern DF: The biology of erbB-2/neu/HER-2 and its role in cancer. Biochim Biophys Acta Rev Cancer 1994;1198:165–184.

Hynes NE: Amplification and overexpression of the erbB-2 gene in human tumors: its involvement in tumor development, significance as a prognostic factor, and potential as a target for cancer therapy. Semin Cancer Biol 1993;4:19–26.

Jarvinen TA, Tanner M, Rantanen V, Barlund M, Borg A, Grenman S, Isola J: Amplification and deletion of topoisomerase IIalpha associate with ErbB-2 amplification and affect sensitivity to topoisomerase II inhibitor doxorubicin in breast cancer. Am J Pathol 2000:156;839–847.

Leitzel K, Teramoto Y, Konrad K, Chinchilli VM, Volas G, Grossberg H, Harvey H, Demers L, Lipton A: Elevated serum c-erbB-2 antigen levels and decreased response to hormone therapy of breast cancer. J Clin Oncol 1995;13:1129–1135.

Leyland-Jones B, Smith I: Role of Herceptin® in primary breast cancer: Views from North America and Europe. Oncology 2001;61 (suppl 2):83–91.

Lipton A, Ali SM, Leitzel K, Chinchilli V, Engle L, Demers L, Brady C, Carney G, Cook B, Cambetas D, Allard J: Elevated serum HER-2/neu level predicts decreased response to hormone therapy in metastatic breast cancer. Proc Am Soc Clin Oncol 2000;19:71A.

Mass RD, Sanders C, Charlene K, Johnson L, Everett T, Anderson S: The concordance between the clinical trials assay (CTA) and fluorescence in situ hybridisation (FISH) in the Herceptin pivotal trials. Proc Am Soc Clin Oncol 2000; 19:75A.

McGuire WL: Breast cancer prognostic factors: evaluation guidelines. J Natl Cancer Inst 1991; 83:1–9.

Ménard S, Valagussa P, Pilotti S, Biganzoli E, Boracchi P, Casalini P, Tomasic G, Marubini E, Colnaghi MI, Cascinelli N, Bonadonna G: Benefit of CMF treatment in lymph node-positive breast cancer overexpressing HER2. Proc Am Soc Clin Oncol 1999;18:69A.

Miles DW, Harris WH, Gillett CE, Smith P, and Barnes DM. Effect of c-erbB(2) and estrogen receptor status on survival in women with primary breast cancer treated with adjuvant cyclophosphamide/methotrexate/fluorouracil. Int J Cancer 1999;84:354–359.

Nordenskjold B, Carstensen J, Rutqvist L, Stal O, Malmstrom P, Ferno M, Borg A, Bergh J, Bengtsson N, Hatschek T, Wallgren A: Prolonged follow-up of the Swedish randomized trial of two versus five years of adjuvant tamoxifen for postmenopausal early stage breast cancer and relationships to hormone receptor and ERBB2 levels. Proc Am Soc Clin Oncol 2000; 19:72A.

Norton L, Slamon D, Leyland-Jones B, Wolter J, Fleming T, Eirmann W, Baselga J, Mendelsohn J, Bajamonde A, Ash M, Shak S: Overall survival (OS) advantage to Herceptin (H) in HER2-overexpressing (HER2+) metastatic breast cancer (MBC). Proc Am Soc Clin Oncol 1999;18:127A.

Paik S, Bryant J, Park C, Fisher B, Tan-Chiu E, Hyams D, Fisher ER, Lippman ME, Wickerham DL, Wolmark N: Erb-B2 and response to doxorubicin in patients with axillary lymph node-positive, hormone-receptor-negative breast cancer. J Natl Cancer Inst 1998;90: 1361–1370.

Pauletti G, Godolphin W, Press MF, Slamon DJ: Detection and quantitation of HER-2/neu gene amplification in human breast cancer archival material using fluorescence in situ hybridization. Oncogene 1996;13:63–72.

Petit T, Ghnassia J, Rodier J, Borel C, Escande A, Mors R, Janser J, Haegelé P: Relationship between erbB-2 status and neoadjuvant chemotherapy response is dependent on anthracycline dose intensity. Proc Am Soc Clin Oncol 2000;19:96A.

Piccart M, Awada A, Hamilton A: Integration of new therapies into management of metastatic breast cancer: a focus on chemotherapy, treatment selection through use of molecular markers, and newly developed biologic therapies in late clinical development. Am Soc Clin Oncol 1999; 35th Annual Meeting, May 15–18, Atlanta, GA. Educational Book 526–39.

Piccart MJ, Di Leo A, Hamilton A: HER2: a 'predictive factor' ready to use in the daily management of breast cancer patients? Eur J Cancer 2000;36:1755–1761.

Ravdin PM, Green S, Albain KS, Boucher V, Ingle J, Pritchard K, Shepard L, Davidson N, Hayes DF, Clark GM, Martino S, Osborne CK, Allred DC: Initial report of the SWOG biological correlative study of C-erbB-2 expression as a predictor of outcome in a trial comparing adjuvant CAF T with tamoxifen (T) alone. Proc Am Soc Clin Oncol 1998;17:97A.

Ries LAG, Kosary CL, Hankey BF, Miller BA, Clegg L, Edwards BK (eds): SEER Cancer Statistics Review, 1973–1996. Bethesda, National Cancer Institute, 1999.

Ross JS, Fletcher JA: The HER-2/neu oncogene in breast cancer: prognostic factor, predictive factor, and target for therapy. Stem Cells 1998;16: 413–428.

Slamon DJ, Clark GM, Wong SG, Levin WJ, Ullrich A, McGuire WL: Human breast cancer: correlation of relapse and survival with amplification of the HER-2/neu oncogene. Science 1987;235:177–182.

Slamon DJ, Godolphin W, Jones LA, Holt JA, Wong SG, Keith DE, Levin WJ, Stuart SG, Udove J, Ullrich A: Studies of the HER-2/neu proto-oncogene in human breast and ovarian cancer. Science 1989;244:707–712.

Slamon D, Leyland-Jones B, Shak S, Paton V, Bajamonde A, Fleming T, Eiermann W, Wolter J, Baselga J, Norton L: Addition of Herceptin™ (humanized anti-HER2 antibody) to first-line chemotherapy for HER2 overexpressing metastatic breast cancer (HER2+/MBC) markedly increases anticancer activity: a randomized, multinational controlled phase III trial. Proc Am Soc Clin Oncol 1998;17:98A.

Slamon D: N Eng J Med 2001, in press.

Stål O, Sullivan S, Wingren S, Skoog L, Rutqvist LE, Carstensen JM, Nordenskjold B: c-erbB2 expression and benefit from adjuvant chemotherapy and radiotherapy of breast cancer. Eur J Cancer 1995;31A:2185–2190.

Thor AD, Berry DA, Budman DR, Muss HB, Kute T, Henderson IC, Barcos M, Cirrincione C, Edgerton S, Allred C, Norton L, Liu ET: Erb-B2, p53 and efficacy of adjuvant therapy in lymph node-positive breast cancer. J Natl Cancer Inst 1998;90:1346–1360.

van de Vijver MJ, Peterse JL, Mooi WJ, Wisman P, Lomans J, Dalesio O, Nusse R: Neu-protein overexpression in breast cancer. Association with comedo-type ductal carcinoma and limited prognostic value in Stage II breast cancer. N Engl J Med 1988;319:1239–1245.

Vogel C, Cobleigh M, Tripathy D, Harris L, Fehrenbacher L, Slamon D, Ash M, Novotny W, Stewart S, Shak S: First-line, non-hormonal, treatment of women with HER2 overexpressing metastatic breast cancer with Herceptin (trastuzumab, humanized anti-HER2 antibody). Proc Am Soc Clin Oncol 2000;19:71A.

Vona G, Caldini A, Sestini R, Rapi S, Bianchi S, Fanelli A, Pazzagli M, Orlando C: The c-erbB-2 oncogene amplification by competitive PCR in aneuploid cell clones flow sorted from breast cancer samples. Clin Chem Lab Med 1999;37: 649–654.

Wright C, Nicholson S, Angus B, Sainsbury JF, Farndon J, Cairns J, Harris AL, Horne CH: Relationship between c-erbB-2 protein product expression and response to endocrine therapy in advanced breast cancer. Br J Cancer 1992; 65:118–121.

Yamauchi H, O'Neill A, Gelman R, Carney W, Tenney DY, Hosch S, Hayes DF: Prediction of response to antiestrogen therapy in advanced breast cancer patients by pretreatment circulating levels of extracellular domain of the HER-2/c-neu protein. J Clin Oncol 1997;15:2518–2525.

Oncology

Oncology 2001;61(suppl 2):83–91

Role of Herceptin® in Primary Breast Cancer: Views from North America and Europe

Brian Leyland-Jones[a] Ian Smith[b]

[a]Department of Oncology, McGill University, Montreal, Canada, [b]Royal Marsden Hospital, Sutton, UK

Key Words
Herceptin® · Trastuzumab · Primary breast cancer · Adjuvant therapy · HER2 · Clinical trials · Neoadjuvant therapy

Abstract
Current therapeutic strategies for primary breast cancer aim to provide improvements in outcome with minimal toxicity to the patient. However, annual relapse rates of up to 12 to 13% during the first 10 years after treatment are seen, and although toxicity has been reduced, it remains a problem in a patient population that is largely asymptomatic. Thus, there is a clear need for more effective therapies. Amplification/overexpression of the human epidermal growth factor receptor-2 (HER2) is an early event in the development of a significant proportion of breast tumors. This abnormality has been shown to have a detrimental effect on prognosis, may predict the outcome of therapies such as tamoxifen and anthracyclines, and provides a target for the novel therapy, Herceptin®. Herceptin is effective and well tolerated in the metastatic setting, making it an ideal candidate for use in adjuvant breast cancer therapy. This has led to the design of a number of trials that aim to provide conclusive evidence as rapidly as possible that Herceptin is well tolerated and effective in the adjuvant setting while also addressing the question of which regimen provides greatest benefit. This review describes these trials and explains how differences in practice between North America and Europe have influenced trial design.

Introduction

The Early Breast Cancer Trialists' Collaborative Group has established that adjuvant polychemotherapy, particularly that involving an anthracycline, reduces the risk of recurrence of primary breast cancer and improves mortality rates in women aged less than 70 years regardless of prognostic status [Early Breast Cancer Trialists' Collaborative Group 1998a]. This same group and others have also shown that hormonal therapy produces benefits in this setting [Early Breast Cancer Trialists' Collaborative Group 1998b; Lønning 2000] and that adding hormonal therapy to chemotherapy produces additional benefits [Early Breast Cancer Trialists' Collaborative Group 1998a, b]. Furthermore, Extermann and colleagues [2000] have reported that in patients aged 65 to 85 years, adjuvant therapy produces reductions in the risk of relapse similar to those observed in younger patients.

Despite these findings, annual breast cancer recurrence rates are as high as 12 to 13% during the first 3 years

KARGER

Fax + 41 61 306 12 34
E-Mail karger@karger.ch
www.karger.com

0030–2414/01/0616–0083$17.50/0

Accessible online at:
www.karger.com/journals/ocl

I. Smith, MD
Royal Marsden Hospital
Downs Road, Sutton
Surrey SM2 5PT (UK)
Tel. +44 181 642 6011, Fax +44 181 643 0373, E-Mail ians@icr.ac.uk

after surgery and appear to stabilize at around 4.5% between 5 and 10 years post-surgery [Saphner et al. 1996]. Therefore, efforts to investigate the potential adjuvant use of novel therapies introduced in the metastatic setting continue [Hortobagyi 2000]. However, it is widely believed that the full benefits of both existing chemotherapeutic agents and hormonal therapies have not yet been realized [Lønning 2000; Piccart et al. 2000a].

Primary breast cancer presents therapeutic challenges that are different from those associated with metastatic disease. Many women with primary breast cancer will have undergone surgery to remove tumors in the breast and axillary lymph nodes and will be asymptomatic. This makes the decision to undergo chemotherapy, which is often debilitating and can cause long-term damage to health, difficult. For this reason, therapies that have relatively few side effects are attractive in the adjuvant setting, and hormonal agents such as tamoxifen and the third-generation aromatase inhibitors have an important role in this regard [Wiseman and Goa 1996; Lønning 2000]. Other considerations include the importance of the dose intensity of cyclophosphamide, methotrexate, 5-fluorouracil (CMF) and anthracyclines [Piccart et al. 2001], lack of benefit of dose escalation above certain doses [Fisher et al. 1997; Bergh et al. 1999; Lotz et al. 1999; Peters et al. 1999] and evidence that estrogen receptor (ER)-negative, progesterone receptor-positive patients obtain benefit from hormonal therapy similar to that of ER-positive patients [Elledge et al. 2000].

Herceptin is well tolerated in the metastatic setting, whether used as a single agent or in combination with chemotherapy [Baselga 1999; Cobleigh et al. 1999; Osoba and Burchmore 1999], with cardiac safety and rare serious infusion-related reactions being the main concerns [Cook-Bruns 2001]. However, the incidence of cardiac events can be minimized with appropriate patient selection and such events have been shown to be manageable [Cobleigh et al. 1999; Cook-Bruns 2001]. The serious infusion reactions observed to date have occurred predominantly in women with extensive lung metastases [Cook-Bruns 2001], which are obviously not a concern in primary breast cancer. In addition to its safety profile, Herceptin has significant efficacy in metastatic disease and the benefits of therapy appear to increase when Herceptin is used earlier rather than later in the course of therapy [Cobleigh et al. 1999; Norton et al. 1999; Burstein et al. 2000; Vogel et al. 2000].

In addition to the known efficacy and tolerability of Herceptin in metastatic breast cancer, a number of other factors make it a good candidate for use as adjuvant therapy. HER2, the tumor target for Herceptin, has been widely reported to have prognostic value [for a review, see Ross and Fletcher 1998]. The increased aggressiveness of tumors in which HER2 is amplified and/or overexpressed [Slamon et al. 1987, 1989] appears to be due to the recognized role of HER2 in increasing the tumorigenicity of cells in which it is amplified and/or overexpressed [Benz et al. 1992; Chazin et al. 1992]. As HER2 overexpression/amplification is an early event in the development of breast cancer [Stark et al. 2000], it would be logical to target this abnormality as soon as possible in the disease process. Another feature of HER2 is that it may predict response to a variety of chemotherapeutic and hormonal agents [for a review, see Piccart 2001]. These two features of HER2 may have value in individualizing therapy in the adjuvant setting, allowing women at high risk of progression to be treated both optimally and aggressively while those at lower risk can be managed more conservatively. Furthermore, they indicate that Herceptin is likely to have clinical value in the treatment of primary breast cancer.

Given that Herceptin has potential in the adjuvant setting, the issue that needs to be addressed is how to establish the optimal method of use so as to maximize efficacy but minimize side effects. Clinical trial design in the adjuvant setting has historically been a problem. Many small studies have produced conflicting results that often overlooked the heterogeneity of breast cancer, and the value of adjuvant therapy took 20 years to establish [Early Breast Cancer Trialists' Collaborative Group 1998a; Piccart-Gebhart 1999]. Thus, large, well-designed adjuvant trials with rapid accrual are needed to establish whether Herceptin provides significant benefit over existing therapies, to identify those patients who will benefit most and to properly elucidate its side-effect profile. This review describes the clinical trial programs that are being established in North America and Europe with the objective of introducing Herceptin into the adjuvant setting. The differences in current practice and how they have affected trial design are also discussed.

View from North America

Although Herceptin has been developed relatively rapidly, it has already been investigated in the metastatic setting in a variety of combinations, at different disease stages and using various dose schedules [Burstein et al. 2000; Cobleigh et al. 1999; Norton et al. 1999; Seidman et al. 2000; Vogel et al. 2000]. The current challenge is to translate the results of these different studies into an adjuvant regimen that provides maximum benefit from Herceptin-containing therapy.

In North America, adjuvant therapy for breast cancer is relatively standardized, with most patients receiving anthracyclines plus cyclophosphamide (currently doxorubicin because epirubicin has only recently been approved) followed by paclitaxel. This is based on data reported by Henderson et al. [1998] showing that this strategy improves both disease-free and overall survival compared with the use of anthracyclines plus cyclophosphamide (AC) alone. Although questions remain regarding the benefit of this strategy, especially in estrogen receptor (ER)-positive patients, the participation of most major institutions in Intergroup trials operated by the National Cancer Institute means that this strategy is widely used. This strategy has also been taken into consideration in the development of Herceptin adjuvant trials. However, the use of platinum analogues in adjuvant breast cancer treatment is also being investigated based on preclinical studies demonstrating synergy [Pietras et al. 1998; Pegram et al. 1999] and clinical studies indicating efficacy [Pegram et al. 1998].

Trials in Metastatic Breast Cancer Supporting the Planned Introduction of Herceptin in the Adjuvant Setting

The rationale for examining these combinations in the adjuvant setting will be based on the results of trials that are currently underway in the metastatic setting. The first of these trials will examine whether carboplatin adds to the benefit of paclitaxel plus Herceptin as first-line therapy for metastatic breast cancer (principal investigators D.J. Slamon, N.J. Robert). This is a multicenter registration trial with an enrolment target of 192 women with metastatic disease who are HER2 2+ or 3+ on immunohistochemistry (IHC), positive by fluorescence in situ hybridization (FISH) or show elevated serum HER2 (sHER2) levels on enzyme-linked immunosorbent assay (ELISA). Patients will receive 3-weekly paclitaxel plus Herceptin according to the standard regimen (4 mg/kg initial dose plus 2 mg/kg weekly) and will then be randomized to 3-weekly carboplatin or no therapy. Similarly, the Breast Cancer International Research Group (BCIRG) is investigating the effect of Herceptin plus docetaxel plus cisplatin or carboplatin in two pilot trials with the aim of studying this regimen in large primary and metastatic breast cancer trials.

A further trial will determine the optimal schedule of paclitaxel and carboplatin for use in combination with Herceptin. This North Central Cancer Treatment Group (NCCTG 98-32-52) trial will randomize women with metastatic breast cancer that is IHC 3+, FISH positive or sHER2 positive to paclitaxel plus carboplatin every 3 weeks or paclitaxel plus carboplatin every week for 3 of 4 weeks, both for six cycles. All patients will receive weekly Herceptin until disease progression. Finally, an Eastern Cooperative Oncology Group trial (E3198) is examining the use of liposomal doxorubicin (Doxil®) as an alternative to doxorubicin. The 200 patients enrolled into this trial will receive liposomal doxorubicin plus docetaxel with or without Herceptin depending on their HER2 status. Together with results that have already been reported, these trials should provide sufficient data to demonstrate which regimens and agents represent the standard of care.

North American Trials of Herceptin in the Adjuvant Setting

The cooperative group network in North America has established a number of large adjuvant breast cancer trials incorporating Herceptin. A major National Surgical Adjuvant Breast and Bowel Project (NSABP) trial is addressing the treatment strategy of AC followed by 3-weekly paclitaxel with or without Herceptin in 2,900 node-positive, HER2-overexpressing breast cancer patients (NSABP B-31). Patients in this trial will receive 4 cycles of 3-weekly AC, before being randomized to 4 cycles of 3-weekly paclitaxel with or without 52 weeks of weekly Herceptin (fig. 1). All drugs will be administered at standard doses. The primary aims are to compare the cardiotoxicity and efficacy in terms of survival of these two regimens, with the effect on disease-free survival as a secondary aim.

An Intergroup study (N9831) will employ the same AC stem as the NSABP trial, but will then randomize patients to weekly paclitaxel × 12, weekly paclitaxel × 12 followed by 52 weeks of Herceptin or weekly paclitaxel plus Herceptin × 12 followed by Herceptin for 40 weeks (fig. 2). This study will provide valuable information on the impact of a paclitaxel dose schedule on outcome as well as the effect on cardiotoxicity of delaying Herceptin administration until 12 weeks after AC administration. The primary endpoints of this trial are disease-free survival and cardiotoxicity, with overall survival, the prognostic value of sHER2 and sHER1, and the concordance of IHC (HercepTest®) and FISH (PathVysion™) and their correlation with outcome as secondary objectives.

The BCIRG preparatory program described above is a prelude to a major international study (BCIRG 006)

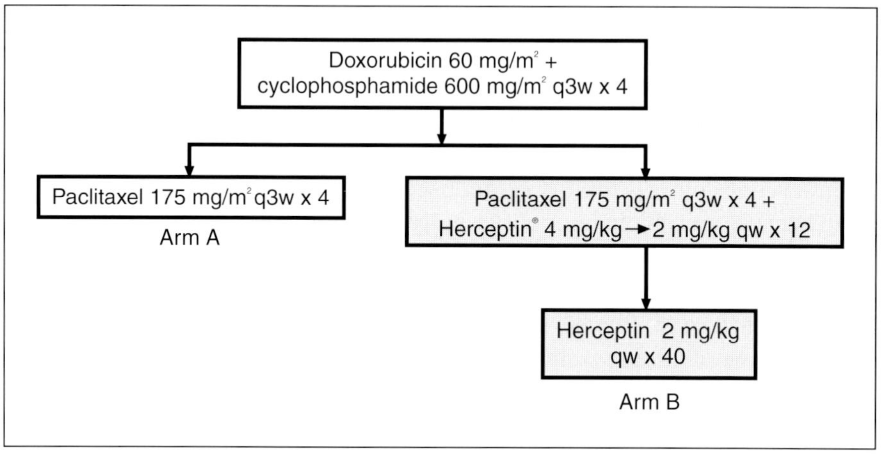

Fig. 1. Design of trial NSABP B-31 in women with node-positive, HER2-positive breast cancer.

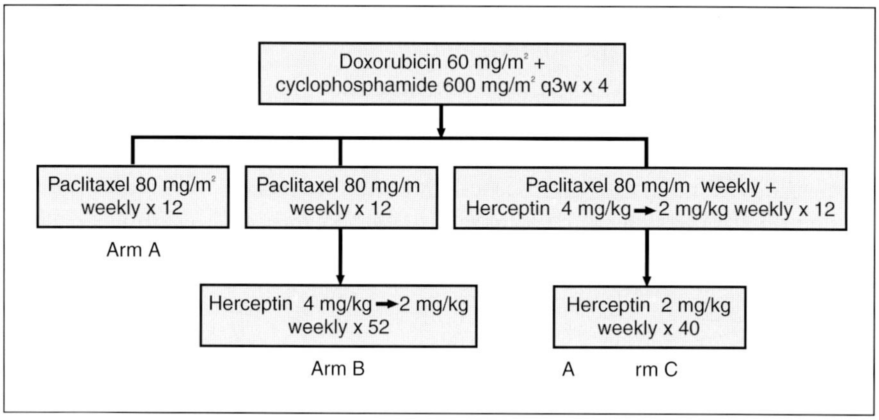

Fig. 2. Design of Intergroup trial N9831 in women with node-positive, HER2-positive breast cancer.

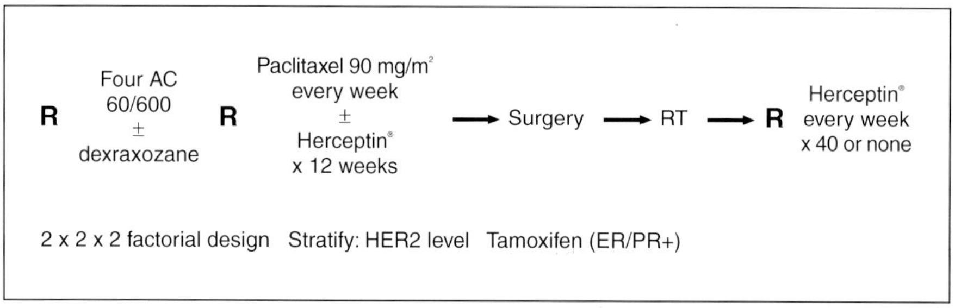

Fig. 3. Design of the Intergroup trial of Herceptin in stage III/inflammatory breast cancer.

incorporating platinum analogs. A total of 2,925 women with node-positive or high-risk node-negative (tumor size ≥2 cm) breast cancer that is HER2 positive by FISH will be enrolled. These patients will be randomized to receive AC followed by docetaxel, AC followed by docetaxel plus Herceptin, or docetaxel, cisplatin/carboplatin plus Herceptin. Disease-free survival is again the primary endpoint.

North American Trials of Herceptin in Locally Advanced Breast Cancer

Studies in locally advanced breast cancer are of interest because they provide a unique opportunity for serial biopsy/evaluations related to the timing of chemotherapy and surgery. The first of these is an Intergroup study originally developed by the Cancer and Leukemia Group B (CALGB) that has a 2 × 2 × 2 factorial design. Patients will be initially randomized to AC × 4 with or without dexrazoxane and then to weekly paclitaxel with or without Herceptin for 12 weeks (fig. 3). Following surgery and radiotherapy, patients will be further randomized to weekly Herceptin for 40 weeks or no therapy. This design will address three issues: whether dexrazoxane can reduce the cardiotoxicity of doxorubicin, whether Herceptin produces benefit in this setting and whether delaying Herceptin administration after AC affects cardiac safety.

A second trial being conducted by the NCCTG will assess the liposomal doxorubicin formulation TLC-D99 plus cyclophosphamide plus Herceptin prior to surgery for locally advanced disease. Surgery will be followed by paclitaxel plus Herceptin for 12 weeks. The endpoints of this trial are pathological complete response, cardiac tolerability and the role of the phosphorylated HER2 receptor in breast cancer.

Summary

The five North American trials of Herceptin in adjuvant and locally advanced breast cancer all incorporate the widely accepted standard treatment stem of AC followed by a taxane, usually paclitaxel. Furthermore, these are large studies that will produce results that that will allow Herceptin to be incorporated into adjuvant therapy as early as possible, although the focus of the BCIRG trials is directed towards the establishment of a docetaxel plus platinum stem. However, they will not provide information on how Herceptin should be incorporated in regions where regimens other than AC followed by a taxane are still widely used. Europe is one such region.

View from Europe

In Europe, the reluctance to accept that adding taxanes to AC is the best regimen in the adjuvant setting is based on clinical trial data as well as national differences. For example, Thomas et al. [2000] recently reported that adding taxanes to AC may not produce a significant improvement in survival. However, definitive proof that AC followed by taxanes is not the optimal strategy is not yet available. In addition, a survey by the Breast International Group [M. Piccart, A. Goldhirsch, personal correspondence] has revealed that there are at least 20 groups performing clinical trials in Europe. These groups are conducting more than 80 trials employing more than 25 schedules, with themes that include anthracyclines versus other chemotherapy, dose-intense or high-dose therapy, and taxane- and vinorelbine-based therapy.

Given the substantial variation in adjuvant practice across Europe, designing European adjuvant trials of Herceptin to provide information that is as useful as possible

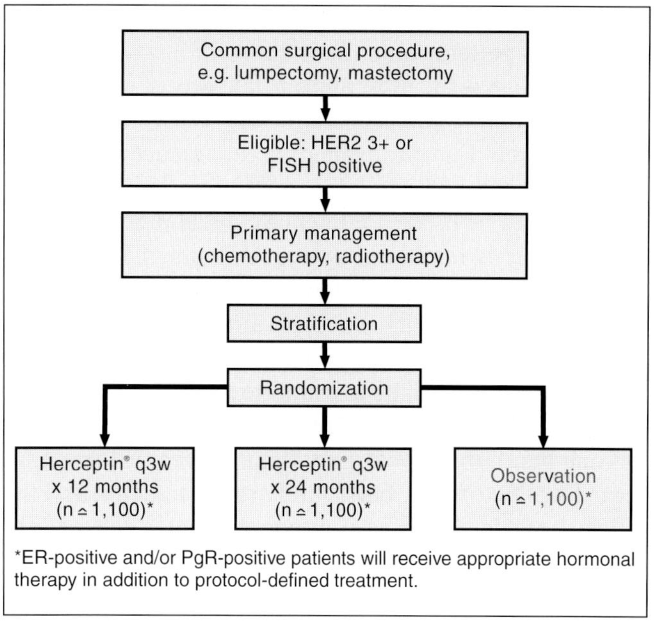

Fig. 4. Design of the HERA Trial (Herceptin Adjuvant Trial) for the treatment of primary breast cancer.

presents a real challenge. Any trials performed must take into account the following issues specifically relating to Herceptin: (1) which patients are eligible for therapy; (2) which chemotherapy regimen should be tested; (3) when should Herceptin be administered in relation to chemotherapy, for how long and which schedule should be used; and (4) whether ER-positive patients should receive tamoxifen.

HERA Trial (Herceptin Adjuvant Trial)

A major international trial of Herceptin as part of adjuvant therapy for approximately 3,300 HER2-positive women with metastatic breast cancer has been designed. Following primary management (chemotherapy, radiotherapy), patients will be randomized to receive 6 mg/kg 3-weekly Herceptin (8 mg/kg initial dose), either for one or two years, or observation (fig. 4). An improvement in disease-free survival is the primary endpoint. Eligibility for trial entry will require HER2 positivity defined as IHC 3+ HER2 overexpression or HER2 gene amplification on FISH testing. This selection process is based on the European indication for Herceptin, which is currently restricted to IHC 3+ patients, and data showing the high level of concordance between outcomes in IHC 3+ and FISH-positive patients [Mass et al. 2000]. The decision to allow the use of any standard or trial chemotherapy regimen is believed to be the best way of recruiting sufficient numbers of patients onto the trial.

This design is the most appropriate way of meeting the objectives, taking into account the differences in adjuvant therapy across Europe, evaluating the impact of Herceptin on outcomes in the adjuvant setting and providing data that can be used to influence clinical practice. However, questions remain even with this pragmatic design. The first is whether to randomize before or after chemotherapy, both of which have advantages and disadvantages in terms of physician and patient bias. The second is whether it is appropriate to examine the issue of not using adjuvant chemotherapy prior to Herceptin in this trial. On one hand, this would provide important information regarding the toxicity, particularly cardiotoxicity, and the efficacy of Herceptin in a previously untreated patient population. On the other hand, however, this would complicate data analysis and reduce the power of the trial. Third, there is no consensus as to how long after chemotherapy and/or radiotherapy Herceptin should be initiated and there are no data to indicate what interval would be optimal. Finally, the 3-weekly Herceptin dose schedule currently being investigated is particularly attractive for use in the adjuvant setting. Recent data have shown this regimen to be promising in metastatic disease [Leyland-Jones et al. 2000a, b].

Other Potential European Trials of Herceptin as Adjuvant Therapy

As discussed above, there are a number of possible agents that could be examined in combination with Herceptin, with vinorelbine and CMF perhaps being particularly appropriate for study in Europe. However, possibly the most interesting combination is that of Herceptin plus tamoxifen. Tamoxifen is widely used in adjuvant therapy for breast cancer because it has been shown to reduce disease recurrence [Early Breast Cancer Trialists' Collaborative Group 1998b] and is well tolerated with few side effects. However, the benefit of adjuvant tamoxifen in the approximately 50% of patients who are ER positive and HER2 positive is uncertain and one trial with extended follow-up has suggested that it may be detrimental [Bianco et al. 2000]. As there is preclinical data to suggest that Herceptin may be able to reverse this resistance [Witters et al. 1997; Kunisue et al. 2000], it is an important concept to investigate clinically.

The best approach to conducting a trial of Herceptin plus tamoxifen is not resolved. Difficulties lie in informing patients that they will receive a potentially detrimental therapy and in obtaining sufficient patient numbers. However, the neoadjuvant setting might prove a suitable route. In a trial comparing neoadjuvant tamoxifen with aromatase inhibitors, 11 of 97 patients were ER positive and HER2 positive [M. Dowsett, I. Smith, unpublished data]. Initial tumor-cell proliferation rates were higher in HER2-positive relative to HER2-negative patients. Interestingly, after 12 weeks of hormonal therapy, the proliferation rates in HER2-positive, ER-positive patients remained higher than those in HER2-negative, ER-positive patients at baseline. Furthermore, data obtained after 2 weeks of therapy were predictive of this difference in response to therapy. Therefore, the effect of adding Herceptin to hormonal therapy could be assessed in a neoadjuvant therapy trial in which patients were randomized to tamoxifen or tamoxifen plus Herceptin for 2 weeks, followed by tamoxifen plus Herceptin for 10 weeks. Measuring proliferation rates at 2 weeks would provide indirect data on the efficacy of adding Herceptin to tamoxifen, while the 10-week extension period would allow response rates to be determined and compared with those in other trials of hormonal therapy alone. This trial design might not produce data as strong as that from an adjuvant study, but is practical and overcomes some of the problems of designing an adjuvant study of Herceptin plus hormonal therapy.

Summary

Adjuvant trials of Herceptin need to be large and pragmatically designed in order to produce answers to questions regarding how to incorporate Herceptin into this setting as quickly as possible. The current European trial design addresses this need and the continuing doubts among European clinicians regarding whether the regimen of AC followed by a taxane is the optimal treatment in the adjuvant setting. The potential to investigate the safety of using Herceptin after a variety of different chemotherapeutic agents and perhaps in patients with no exposure to chemotherapy may also produce vital data. Finally, the use of a neoadjuvant trial of Herceptin in combination with hormonal therapy to produce evidence applicable to the adjuvant setting is a novel method of examining a difficult question.

Conclusions

The need for more effective therapies for primary breast cancer is overwhelming despite evidence that anthracyclines have improved outcomes in this population, that adding hormonal therapy to chemotherapy further

Table 1. Summary of trials of Herceptin in primary breast cancer

Study	Details	Endpoints
North America		
NSABP B-31	Randomized trial of AC followed by paclitaxel or paclitaxel + Herceptin in node-positive, HER2-positive women	Overall survival, cardiac safety
N9831	Randomized trial of AC followed by paclitaxel, paclitaxel followed by Herceptin, or paclitaxel + Herceptin in node-positive, HER2-positive women	Disease-free survival, cardiac safety
BCIRG 006	Randomized trial of AC followed by docetaxel, docetaxel + Herceptin, or docetaxel + cisplatin/carboplatin + Herceptin in node-positive and high-risk node-negative, HER2-positive women	Disease-free survival
Intergroup study in stage III/ inflammatory breast cancer	2 × 2 × 2 factorial design in which women will be randomized to AC ± dexrazoxane, followed by paclitaxel ± Herceptin followed by surgery and radiotherapy ± Herceptin	Pathological complete response, cardiac safety
NCCTG study in locally advanced breast cancer	Randomized phase II trial of TLC-D99 + cyclophosphamide + Herceptin followed by surgery and paclitaxel + Herceptin	Pathological complete response, cardiac safety
Europe		
HERA Trial (Herceptin Adjuvant Trial)	Randomized trial comparing 1 or 2 years of Herceptin with no Herceptin in patients who have completed adjuvant chemotherapy	Improvement in disease-free survival
Neoadjuvant study of tamoxifen ± Herceptin	Randomized trial of tamoxifen ± Herceptin for 2 weeks followed by tamoxifen + Herceptin for 10 weeks followed by surgery	Tumour proliferation rate, response rate

reduces relapse rates and that a regimen of AC followed by a taxane may provide additional benefit. Therapies that are better tolerated than current regimens while having proven efficacy in high-risk patient groups are particularly important. The humanized anti-HER2 monoclonal antibody, Herceptin, has proven efficacy in a high-risk patient population with metastatic breast cancer: HER2-positive patients have been shown to have significantly reduced disease-free and overall survival. These features, coupled with the known role of HER2 in oncogenicity throughout the disease course in breast cancer patients and the observed safety profile of Herceptin, make this agent an ideal candidate for study in the treatment of primary breast cancer.

Adjuvant studies of Herceptin that are planned in North America and Europe will address a number of fundamental questions regarding the efficacy and safety of the drug. Despite differences in standard care for patients with primary breast cancer between these two regions, these studies benefit from good design, being powered to reliably identify variations between treatment regimens and the inclusion of most of the major chemotherapy regimens currently in clinical use (table 1). This pragmatic and coordinated approach that is made possible through the use of the US cooperative group system, the BCIRG and a pan-European investigator group should provide data on the best use of Herceptin in the adjuvant setting in the shortest possible time. Based on survival data obtained for Herceptin in the treatment of metastatic disease and experience with other therapies that have moved from the metastatic to the adjuvant setting, it is predicted that Herceptin will have a significant positive impact on survival in patients with primary breast cancer.

References

Baselga J: Safety profile of Herceptin (R) as a single agent and in combination with chemotherapy. Eur J Cancer 1999;35(suppl 4):S324A.

Benz CC, Scott GK, Sarup JC, Johnson RM, Tripathy D, Coronado E, Shepard HM, Osborne CK: Estrogen-dependent, tamoxifen-dependent tumorigenic growth of MCF-7 cells transfected with HER2/*neu*. Breast Cancer Res Treat 1992;24:85–95.

Bergh J: Results from a randomized adjuvant breast cancer study with high-dose chemotherapy with CTCb supported by autologous bone marrow stem cells versus dose-escalated and tailored FEC therapy. Proc Am Soc Clin Oncol 1999;18:2A.

Bianco AR, De Laurentiis M, Carlomagno C, Gallo C, Panico L, De Placido S: HER2 overexpression predicts adjuvant tamoxifen (TAM) failure for early breast cancer (EBC): complete data at 20 yr of the Naples GUN randomized trial. Proc Am Soc Clin Oncol 2000;19:75A.

Burstein HJ, Kuter I, Richardson PG, Campos SM, Matulonis UA, Harris L, Garber JE, Younger J, Bunnell CA, Shulman LN, Winer EP: Herceptin (H) and Navelbine (V) for HER2-positive metastatic breast cancer: a phase II study. Proc Am Soc Clin Oncol 2000;19:102A.

Chazin VR, Kaleko M, Miller AD, Slamon DJ: Transformation mediated by the human HER-2 gene independent of the epidermal growth factor receptor. Oncogene 1992;7:1859–1866.

Cobleigh MA, Vogel CL, Tripathy D, Robert NJ, Scholl S, Fehrenbacher L, Wolter JM, Paton V, Shak S, Lieberman G, Slamon DJ: Multinational study of the efficacy and safety of humanized anti-HER2 monoclonal antibody in women who have HER2-overexpressing metastatic breast cancer that has progressed after chemotherapy for metastatic disease. J Clin Oncol 1999;17:2639–2648.

Cook-Bruns N: Retrospective analysis of the safety of Herceptin® immunotherapy in metastatic breast cancer. Oncology 2001;61(suppl 2):58–66.

Early Breast Cancer Trialists' Collaborative Group: Polychemotherapy for early breast cancer: an overview of the randomised trials. Lancet 1998a;352:930–942.

Early Breast Cancer Trialists' Collaborative Group: Tamoxifen for early breast cancer: an overview of the randomised trials. Lancet 1998b;351:1451–1467.

Elledge RM, Green S, Pugh R, Allred DC, ClarkGM, Hill J, Ravdin P, Martino S, Osborne CK: Estrogen receptor (ER) and progesterone receptor (PgR), by ligand-binding assay compared with ER, PgR and pS2 by immunohistochemistry in predicting response to tamoxifen in metastatic breast cancer: a Southwest Oncology Group Study. Int J Cancer 2000;89:111–117.

Extermann M, Balducci L, Lyman GH: What threshold for adjuvant therapy in older breast cancer patients? J Clin Oncol 2000;18:1709–1717.

Fisher B, Anderson S, Wickerham DL, DeCillis A, Dimitrov N, Mamounas E, Wolmark N, Pugh R, Atkins J, Meyers FJ, Abramson N, Wolter J, Bornstein RS, Levy L, Romond EH, Caggiano V, Grimaldi M, Jochimsen P, Deckers P: Further evaluation of intensified and total dose of cyclophosphamide in a doxorubicin-cyclophosphamide regimen for the treatment of primary breast cancer: Findings from National Surgical Adjuvant Breast and Bowel Project B-22. J Clin Oncol 1997;15:1858–1869.

Henderson IC, Berry D, Demetri G, Cirrincione C, Goldstein L, Martino S, Ingle JN, Cooper MR, Canellos G, Borden E, Fleming G, Holland JF, Graziano S, Carpenter J, Muss H, Norton L, for CALGB, ECOG, SWOG, and NCCTG: Improved disease-free survival (DFS) and overall survival (OS) from the addition of sequential paclitaxel (T) but not from the escalation of doxorubicin (A) dose level in the adjuvant chemotherapy of patients (pts) with node-positive primary breast cancer. Proc Am Soc Clin Oncol 1998;17:101A.

Hortobagyi GN: Developments in chemotherapy of breast cancer. Cancer 2000;88(suppl 12): 3073–3079.

Kunisue H, Kurebayashi J, Otsuki T, Tang CK, Kurosumi M, Yamamoto S, Tanaka K, Doihara H, Shimizu N, Sonoo H: Anti-HER2 antibody enhances the growth inhibitory effect of anti-oestrogen on breast cancer cells expressing both oestrogen receptors and HER2. Br J Cancer 2000;82:46–51.

Leyland-Jones B, Arnold A, Gelmon K, Verma S, Rakhit A, Howell J. A pharmacokinetic (PK) study of Herceptin® administered with paclitaxel i.v. every 3 weeks. Eur J Cancer 2000a; S35:abstract 41.

Leyland-Jones B, Hemmings F, Arnold A, Gelmon K, Verma S, Ayoub J-P. Pharmacokinetics of Herceptin® administered with paclitaxel every three weeks. Cancer Res Treat 2000b;124:abstract 534.

Lønning PE: Is there a growing role for endocrine therapy in the treatment of breast cancer? Drugs 2000;60:11–21.

Lotz JP, Cure H, Janvier M, Morvan F, Asselain B, Guillemot M, Laadem A, Maraninchi D, Gisselbrecht C, Roché H, and the PEGASE Group: High-dose chemotherapy with hematopoietic stem cells transplantation for metastatic breast cancer: Results of the Finnish protocol Pegase 04. Proc Am Soc Clin Oncol 1999;18: 43A.

Mass R, Sanders C, Kasian C, Everett T, Johnson L, Anderson S: The concordance between the Clinical Trials Assay (CTA) and fluorecence in situ hybridization (FISH) in the Herceptin® pivotal trials. Proc Am Soc Clin Oncol 2000; 19:75A.

Norton L, Slamon D, Leyland-Jones B, Wolter J, Fleming T, Eirmann W, Baselga J, Mendelsohn J, Bajamonde A, Ash M, Shak S: Overall survival (OS) advantage to simultaneous chemotherapy (CRx) plus the humanized anti-HER2 monoclonal antibody Herceptin (H) in HER2-overexpressing (HER2+) metastatic breast cancer (MBC). Proc Am Soc Clin Oncol 1999;18: 127A.

Osoba D, Burchmore M: Health-related quality of life in women with metastatic breast cancer treated with trastuzumab (Herceptin). Semin Oncol 1999;26(suppl 12):84–88.

Pegram M, Hsu S, Lewis G, Pietras R, Beryt M, Sliwkowski M, Coombs D, Baly D, Kabbinavar F, Slamon D: Inhibitory effects of combinations of HER-2/*neu* antibody and chemotherapeutic agents used for treatment of human breast cancers. Oncogene 1999;18:2241–2251.

Pegram MD, Lipton A, Hayes DF, Weber BL, Baselga JM, Tripathy D, Baughman SA, Twaddell T, Glaspy JA, Slamon DJ: Phase II study of receptor-enhanced chemosensitivity using recombinant humanized anti-p185$^{\mathrm{HER2}/neu}$ monoclonal antibody plus cisplatin in patients with HER2/*neu*-overexpressing metastatic breast cancer refractory to chemotherapy treatment. J Clin Oncol 1998;16:2659–2671.

Peters WP, Rosner G, Vredenburgh J, Shpall E, Crump M, Richardson P, Marks L, Cirrincione C, Wood W, Henderson I, Hurd D, Norton L: A prospective, randomized comparison of two doses of combination alkylating agents as consolidation after CAF in high-risk primary breast cancer involving ten or more axillary lymph nodes: Preliminary results of CALGB 9082/SWOG 9114/NCIC MA-13. Proc Am Soc Clin Oncol 1999;18:1A.

Piccart M, Lohrisch C, Di Leo A, Larsimont D: The predictive value of HER2 in breast cancer. Oncology 2001;61(suppl 2):73–82.

Piccart MJ, Biganzoli L, Di Leo A: The impact of chemotherapy dose density and dose intensity on breast cancer outcome: what have we learned? Eur J Cancer. 2000b;36(suppl 1):S4–S10.

Piccart MJ, Lohrisch C, Straehle C: New strategies in the treatment of non-metastatic breast cancer. 10th International Congress on Anti-Cancer Treatment Book of Abstracts 2000a:47–49.

Piccart-Gebhart M: What can be expected from the next generation of adjuvant breast cancer treatment? Semin Oncol 1999;26(suppl 3):22–25.

Pietras RJ, Pegram MD, Finn RS, Maneval DA, Slamon DJ: Remission of human breast cancer xenografts on therapy with humanized monoclonal antibody to HER-2 receptor and DNA-reactive drugs. Oncogene 1998;17:2235–2249.

Ross JS, Fletcher JA: The HER-2/*neu* oncogene in breast cancer: prognostic factor, predictive factor, and target for therapy. Stem Cells 1998;16: 413–428.

Saphner T, Tormey DC, Gray R: Annual hazard rates of recurrence for breast cancer after primary therapy. J Clin Oncol 1996;14:2738–2746.

Seidman AD, Formier M, Esteva FJ, Tan L, Kaptain S, Bach A, Panageas K, Arroyo C, Currie V, Gilewski T, Theodoulou M, Moynahan ME, Moasser M, Sklarin N, Dickler M, Chin J, Denton C, Bacotti D, Frye D, Hortobagyi G, Norton L, Hudis C: Final report: weekly Herceptin and Taxol for metastatic breast cancer with analysis of efficacy by HER2 immunophenotype (IHC) and gene amplification (FISH). Proc Am Soc Clin Oncol 2000;19:83A.

Slamon DJ, Clark GM, Wong SG, Levin WJ, Ullrich A, McGuire WL: Human breast cancer: correlation of relapse and survival with amplification of the HER-2/*neu* oncogene. Science 1987;235:177–182.

Slamon DJ, Godolphin W, Jones LA, Holt JA, Wong SG, Keith DE, Levin WJ, Stuart SG, Udove J, Ullrich A: Studies of the HER-2/*neu* proto-oncogene in human breast and ovarian cancer. Science 1989;244:707–712.

Stark A, Hulka BS, Joens S, Novotny D, Thor AD, Wold LE, Schell MJ, Melton III, LJ, Liu ET, Conway K: *HER-2/neu* amplification in benign breast disease and the risk of subsequent breast cancer. J Clin Oncol 2000;18:267–274.

Thomas E, Buzdar A, Theriault R, Singletary S, Booser D, Valero V, Ibrahim N, Smith T, Frye D, Manuel N, Kau S, McNeese M: Role of paclitaxel in adjuvant therapy of operable breast cancer: preliminary results of prospective randomised clinical trial. Proc Am Soc Clin Oncol 2000;19:74A.

Vogel C, Cobleigh M, Tripathy D, Harris L, Fehrenbacher L, Slamon D, Ash M, Novotny W, Stewart S, Shak S: First-line, non-hormonal, treatment of woman with HER2 overexpressing metastatic breast cancer with Herceptin (trastuzumab, humanized anti-HER2 antibody). Proc Am Soc Clin Oncol 2000;19:71A.

Wiseman LR, Goa KL: Formestane: a review of its pharmacological properties and clinical efficacy in the treatment of postmenopausal breast cancer. Drugs Aging 1996;9:292–306.

Witters LM, Kumar R, Chincilli VM, Lipton A: Enhanced anti-proliferative activity of the combination of tamoxifen plus HER-2-neu antibody. Breast Cancer Res Treat 1997;42:1–5.

Oncology

Author Index Vol. 61, Suppl. 2, 2001

Subject Index Vol. 61, Suppl. 2, 2001

KARGER
Fax + 41 61 306 12 34
E-Mail karger@karger.ch
www.karger.com

Accessible online at:
www.karger.com/journals/ocl